THE HASHIMOTO'S AIP COOKBOOK

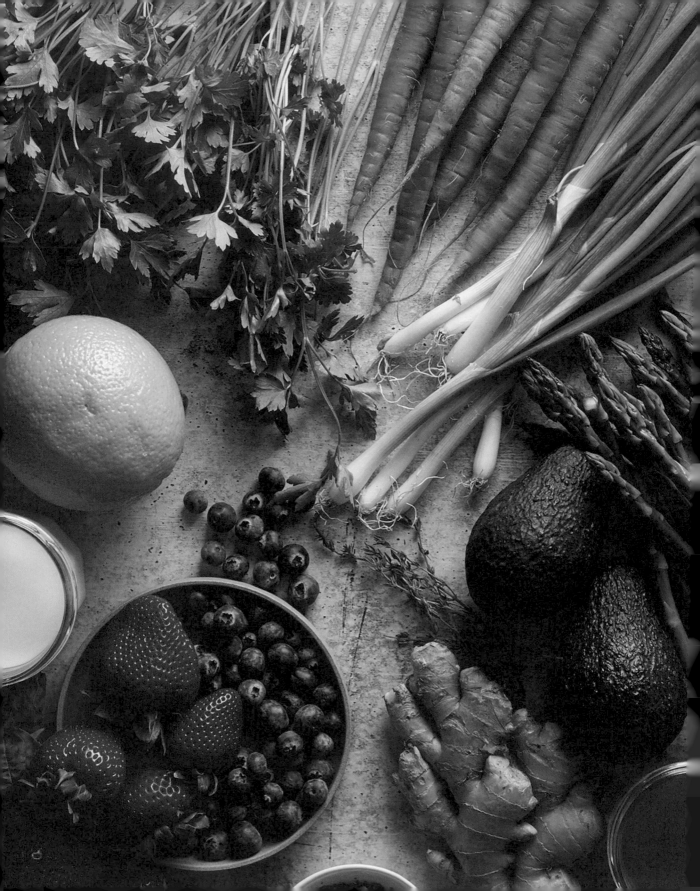

The Hashimoto's AIP Cookbook

Easy Recipes for Thyroid Healing on the Paleo Autoimmune Protocol

Emily Kyle, MS, RDN, CLT, HCP

Phil Kyle, Chef

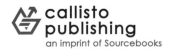

callisto
publishing
an imprint of Sourcebooks

To my "Unkel Judy," and all the men and women who live, survive, and thrive while managing Hashimoto's and other chronic autoimmune conditions.

Copyright © 2019 by Callisto Publishing LLC

Cover and internal design © 2019 by Callisto Publishing LLC

Photography © 2019 Evi Abeler. Food styling by Albane Sharrard.

Author photo courtesy of © Creative Touch Design & Photography.

Interior and Cover Designer: Will Mack

Art Producer: Sara Feinstein

Editor: Clara Song Lee

Production Manager: Riley Hoffman

Production Editor: Melissa Edeburn

Published by Callisto Publishing LLC C/O Sourcebooks LLC

P.O. Box 4410, Naperville, Illinois 60567-4410

(630) 961-3900

callistopublishing.com

Printed and bound in China.

OGP 19

Contents

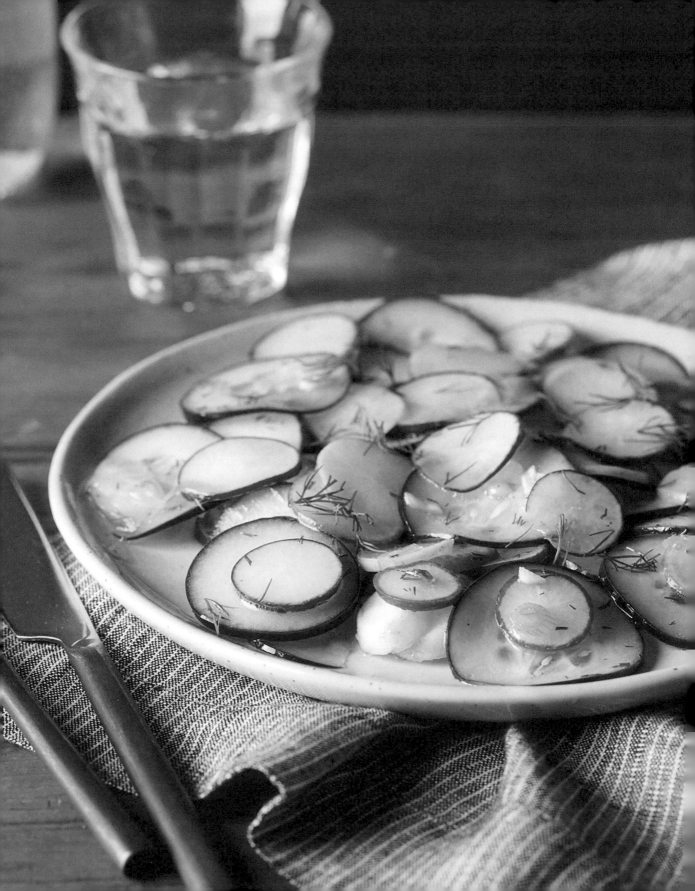

Introduction

*a*fter I wrote my first book, *The 30-Minute Thyroid Cookbook: 125 Healing Recipes for Hypothyroidism and Hashimoto's*, I was taken aback by how many people confided in me that they, too, suffered from Hashimoto's disease in secret.

Hashimoto's thyroiditis affects 14 million people in the United States alone, making it not only the most common form of thyroiditis, but also the most common thyroid disorder in America. Women are seven times more likely than men to be diagnosed with this autoimmune disease, making it an especially important women's health issue facing Americans today.

Yet, it seems that no one is talking about Hashimoto's in an open and honest way.

We tend to hide the impact that negative symptoms have on our everyday lives. We dismiss the fatigue and lethargy, fight through the brain fog and forgetfulness, and constantly battle the uncontrollable weight gain as if it is just a "normal" part of getting older. Many of us don't speak up when we visit our doctors because we don't want to be seen as complainers, or we think the symptoms are normal enough to live with. We don't confide in others because we are afraid of being judged.

Like I tell so many of the clients that I work with in my private practice, you do not have to live the rest of your life feeling unwell. You do not need to live the rest of your life feeling so fatigued that some days you can't get out of bed. You do not need to continually miss family outings and social gatherings because you are too tired to get dressed, let alone leave the house. And you definitely do not need to live the rest of your life feeling like you are alone and isolated in this struggle.

As a registered dietitian nutritionist who provides functional nutrition guidance for my patients suffering from autoimmune and inflammatory conditions, I have found that one of the first steps to addressing the management of Hashimoto's disease is to implement an elimination diet like the paleo autoimmune protocol (also known as AIP), or to participate in food sensitivity testing. I have watched countless patients, after following the protocol, successfully identify and pinpoint their specific dietary triggers, which then leads to many other positive lifestyle changes.

However, I will admit that the AIP may seem daunting. When I wrote my first cookbook, which touched on the AIP, I had a bit more flexibility with the ingredients and the recipes, and I was able to create most of the tasty dishes on my own. When I took on this cookbook, I knew that even with my expertise, I would need guidance to create AIP-compliant food that tasted not just good, but amazing.

I knew I had no choice but to go to my husband and ask for help. As a busy restaurant owner (and smart guy), he generously agreed to help me on this new project. Together, we explored this new collaboration and began to learn from and inspire each other. In the end, we combined the best of our knowledge and expertise to create a cookbook that provides easy, nutrient-dense recipes that really do taste amazing, all while adhering to the AIP. We hope you enjoy these dishes as much as we enjoyed creating them.

My goal with this book is to give you the hope, optimism, encouragement, and guidance you need to start baby-stepping your way into a holistic lifestyle that supports your physical, mental, and emotional health. I want to help you create a physically supportive diet that you can use in partnership with any mental and emotional acts of self-care you do to facilitate healing.

Many conventional medical providers prefer to prescribe medications to their patients without addressing diet and lifestyle interventions. I believe in the immense healing power of food and nutrition. There is no known cure for Hashimoto's disease, but you can take steps to live a healthy, vibrant life and feel well again.

In fact, the majority of people suffering from autoimmune conditions like Hashimoto's see a dramatic reduction in their signs and symptoms in as few as 15 to 30 days with the implementation of the AIP. Those who are truly suffering from an autoimmune condition triggered by hidden food sensitivities find the most relief the quickest.

Through this book, I hope to give you the guidance and resources you need to help heal your body and support optimal thyroid health and immune function with approachable, real-world recipes. I want you to *enjoy* the paleo autoimmune protocol as it helps you find lasting relief from your most challenging symptoms.

Of course, if you struggle with any part of the paleo autoimmune protocol, do not hesitate to reach out to me directly, contact your health care provider, or access the resources listed in the back of this book (page 184) for added support and guidance. You do not need to go through this process alone. Begin to build your support team. Join me on this journey, and together we can begin to reduce your most debilitating symptoms and restore the health and vitality you deserve.

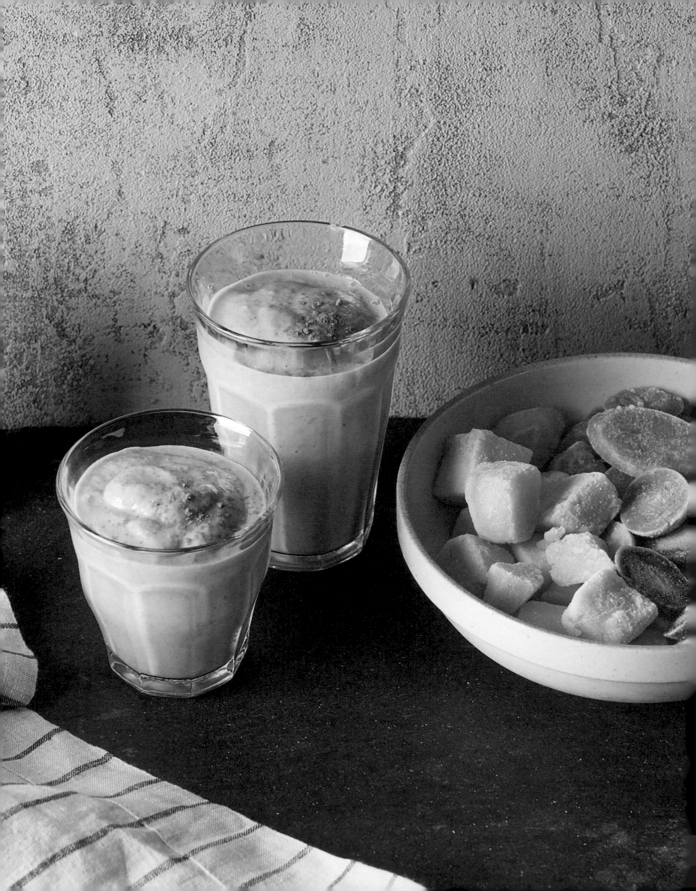

1 *Healing Hashimoto's with the AIP*

Hashimoto's disease is an autoimmune disorder and the leading cause of hypothyroidism, or underactive thyroid. In this chapter, we will explore what is happening in the body on a functional level, the important connection between diet and autoimmune disorders, and how the paleo autoimmune protocol (AIP) may help sufferers of Hashimoto's enough to reduce or even eliminate troublesome symptoms. The AIP is a stricter version of the Paleo diet (see page 6), and it is designed to reduce inflammation, heal the gut, and support overall thyroid health.

THE CONNECTION BETWEEN DIET AND AUTOIMMUNE DISORDERS

Generally speaking, an autoimmune disease is one in which the immune system mistakenly attacks the body. There are many theories about what causes auto-immune disorders; some scientists believe these conditions are a result of the immune system falsely attacking the thyroid gland, whereas others believe they are a result of the immune system falling victim to the Epstein-Barr virus. Regardless of the cause, scientific research confirms the connection between diet and autoimmune disorders. Professionals and patients alike agree that food can have a tremendous impact on the management of autoimmune disorders, and various studies have shown that food has the power to heal the body and alleviate symptoms associated with Hashimoto's and other autoimmune conditions.

Immune System Basics

The immune system is a complex network of cells, proteins, tissues, and organs that work together to protect the body from infection. As our skin is the outside layer of defense for the body, our immune system is the inside layer of defense, detecting and protecting against viruses, bacteria, parasites, fungi, and other potentially dangerous microorganisms.

There are many layers of defense that work together to protect the body against infection and disease, and this is what makes the immune system so complex. Even the immune system can be broken down into subsystems. In a healthy immune system, these systems work together to recognize, neutralize, and fight pathogens that enter the body.

The immune system must know when it has to fight against the body's own cells that may have changed into something potentially dangerous, such as cancerous cells. A properly functioning immune system can differentiate between cells that are from the body and cells that are not, and, more important it can recognize if those cells are helpful or harmful.

If the immune system mistakes healthy cells for foreign or unhealthy cells, it will generate antibodies to fight these healthy cells and tissues, resulting in damage. Over time, this faulty immune response can lead to autoimmune disease.

In the case of Hashimoto's, the body misidentifies the cells that produce the thyroid hormone as foreign invaders, causing an immune response that interferes with the function of the thyroid gland and the production of thyroid hormones.

It is thought that genetic and environmental factors play an important role in the development, onset, and duration of autoimmune diseases.

THE PROBLEM OF LEAKY GUT

Leaky gut is a popular phrase used to describe what the medical community calls "increased intestinal permeability." The intestines have a protective lining that is responsible for preventing antigens, toxins, bacteria, and other pathogens from leaving the intestines and being absorbed into the bloodstream. However, when this intestinal lining is compromised—as a result of environmental factors, heredity, or illness—it begins to allow foreign substances or toxins to escape ("leak") out of the digestive system and into the blood. This phenomenon can promote an immune response that may cause or worsen autoimmune conditions. Diet and lifestyle modifications that protect the gut are an important part of treatment for anyone living with an autoimmune condition.

Hashimoto's Disease

Hashimoto's is an autoimmune condition that occurs when the body's immune system misidentifies and attacks the healthy tissue of the thyroid gland. Over time, this response results in hypothyroidism. According to the American Thyroid Association, hypothyroidism is a condition characterized by an abnormally low level of activity in the thyroid gland, meaning it does not produce enough thyroid hormone to keep the body running properly. Hashimoto's disease is the leading cause of hypothyroidism in America, but not everyone who is diagnosed with Hashimoto's develops hypothyroidism. Hashimoto's thyroiditis involves inflammation of the thyroid gland, usually caused by an autoimmune attack or a viral infection. Over time, this chronic inflammation can damage the thyroid gland and lead to hypothyroidism.

Unfortunately, it is entirely possible to have Hashimoto's without symptoms for a prolonged period, which makes identifying and treating the disease even more difficult. Many people suffer silently for years, thinking that their fatigue, aches, or brain fog are just part of life, unaware that these symptoms are being caused by Hashimoto's. Once the symptoms do finally reveal their connection to the disease, many people find themselves too sick and exhausted to undertake the large task of overhauling their diet and lifestyle to facilitate healing.

Many symptoms of Hashimoto's have a negative impact on both the body and the mind. This impact makes the ever-important process of self-care even more difficult. Many of the symptoms are vague and hard to pinpoint right away; they develop over time with a slow and prolonged attack on the thyroid. Some of the more general symptoms of Hashimoto's include:

- Weight gain
- Fatigue
- Drowsiness
- Brain fog or difficulty concentrating
- Constipation
- Infertility

Some of the more specific symptoms that help identify Hashimoto's disease include:

- Dry hair, skin, and nails
- Unusual hair loss or thinning eyebrows
- Increased sensitivity to the cold
- Puffiness or paleness in the face
- Muscle soreness

Hashimoto's, which is more prevalent in women than in men, presents itself with symptoms that are especially difficult to deal with because they simultaneously affect physical and mental health in a variety of ways. Living in a culture that values thinness over health is especially frustrating for those who are facing stubborn weight loss efforts or, even worse, uncontrollable weight gain. This phenomenon affects both the mental and physical health of individuals who are frustrated with their lack of control over their bodies and their health. Additionally, the brain fog and extreme fatigue associated with Hashimoto's make it very difficult to concentrate on the restoration of health through diet and lifestyle modifications.

When It's More Than Hashimoto's

Autoimmune diseases can co-occur. For example, many people with Hashimoto's suffer from other conditions such as celiac disease or food allergies, and it can be frustrating when diet modifications for these different diagnoses contradict one another, as they often do.

Thankfully, the paleo autoimmune protocol (AIP) is not exclusively for those with Hashimoto's. Though it is one of the most restrictive elimination protocols, AIP is also the most commonly prescribed protocol for autoimmune conditions ranging from celiac disease to rheumatoid arthritis, because it removes the major dietary triggers that can cause inflammation and unwanted reactions in a variety of different disease scenarios.

Although the AIP may be difficult to implement, it can alleviate the need to mesh together two different diets for two different conditions. In many cases, following the AIP may be the quickest and easiest way to address the root cause of many of the symptoms brought on by autoimmune diseases in general.

How Diet Affects Hashimoto's

Addressing the root cause of Hashimoto's symptoms and getting the disease under control are impossible without addressing gut health, which is what a healing, restorative diet can do. Leaky gut is a major problem for those living with Hashimoto's or other autoimmune conditions, and it must be addressed in order to experience true healing. Leaky gut can contribute to the overall diseased state of the body and worsen Hashimoto's symptoms; therefore, a gut-healing dietary protocol is critical. A combination of the right diet and the right lifestyle interventions can help restore thyroid function and minimize or even eliminate common symptoms such as fatigue, hair loss, weight gain, and depression.

At this time, there is no known cure for Hashimoto's, so the main goal of the medical nutrition therapy treatment for this condition is to reduce the level of inflammation in the body and calm the immune response. By working to temper inflammation and heal the lining of the gut through diet and lifestyle interventions, we can begin to manage and treat the symptoms that result from this frustrating condition. Hashimoto's affects every person differently, making the approach to defining an optimal diet for the population nearly impossible—hence the importance of individualized care and diet. A healthy diet that is tailored to an individual's unique needs offers the greatest potential to reduce or even reverse Hashimoto's symptoms.

THE PALEO AUTOIMMUNE PROTOCOL

The paleo autoimmune protocol is a proven approach to wellness, including both dietary and lifestyle modifications. However, for the purpose of this book, we will be focusing primarily on the dietary component.

How the Protocol Works

By eliminating or restricting the most potentially inflammatory foods from the diet, the AIP allows the body to reduce the constant inflammatory response, to promote gut healing, and to rest and recover. After the recovery period, foods are reintroduced one at a time to identify any negative responses. This process allows individuals to get a clear picture of what their specific dietary triggers are, without the need to restrict all major food groups for the long term.

The Paleo diet, from which the AIP is derived, involves a way of eating that may have been similar to that of early hunters and gatherers before the advent of farming practices. It focuses on meat, fruit, vegetables, nuts, and seeds. The stricter AIP (which eliminates nuts and seeds) focuses on consumption of a wide variety of anti-inflammatory foods and avoidance of foods in the following categories (see the complete list on page 20):

- Dairy
- Gluten and grains
- Eggs
- Legumes
- Nightshade vegetables

- Nuts and seeds
- Added sugar
- Food additives, artificial sweeteners, processed vegetable oils
- Alcohol

Remember, the goal of the protocol is not to eliminate these foods from your life forever. By avoiding these foods for a length of time, you are allowing the body to heal and prepare for the reintroduction phase of the protocol. It's also important to remember the long-term payoff for this temporary inconvenience: Studies have shown that following the AIP can help repair leaky gut, alter intestinal permeability, and promote healing from a wide range of autoimmune conditions.

You may be asking, "What can I eat on the AIP?" Good question. During the elimination phase, it is just as important to enjoy meals filled with nourishing, nutrient-dense foods as it is to restrict inflammatory foods. Generally, the following anti-inflammatory foods are allowed during the elimination phase of the protocol (see the complete list on page 20):

- Wild-caught meat and fish
- Vegetables (except nightshades)
- Small quantities of fruit and sweet potatoes
- Coconut milk
- Oils made from avocado, olives, or coconut

- Small quantities of raw honey or pure maple syrup
- Fresh herbs
- Dairy-free fermented foods
- Vinegar
- Herbal teas
- Homemade bone broth

These nutrient-rich, anti-inflammatory foods will help heal the gut and quiet the immune response. They are consumed while foods that are suspected to cause inflammation are eliminated. If the AIP feels restrictive, just remember: Its duration is temporary, but its positive effects are long-lasting.

How temporary? There are two main phases of the AIP: an elimination phase and a reintroduction phase.

During the elimination phase, all of the inflammatory foods are eliminated. This phase should be no shorter than 30 days and typically lasts 60 to 90 days to allow the body adequate time to heal and be nourished.

During the reintroduction phase, foods are added one by one back into the diet, following a specific reintroduction schedule. At the end of this phase, you will have a personalized diet tailored to your own specific health needs.

Considerations for Hashimoto's

The AIP is comprehensive enough on its own to provide necessary dietary relief to those with Hashimoto's, but here are some important nutrients to pay special attention to if you have this condition. Note: Reintroducing foods containing gluten is not recommended. It is widely accepted that all Hashimoto's patients should abstain from gluten-containing foods for the long term.

Iodine An iodine deficiency was once thought to be the sole cause of hypothyroidism, so for a while, iodine supplementation was the standard treatment. Although iodine supplementation may be helpful to some individuals, more recent studies have shown that the disease process is much more complicated and cannot simply be treated by iodine supplementation alone.

Calcium Calcium is critical for supporting both immune and thyroid function. Hypothyroidism can inhibit calcium metabolism and is known to be one of the leading causes of osteoporosis.

Vitamin D According to a study published in the *International Journal of Health Studies* in 2013, the degree and severity of hypothyroidism may be significantly associated with vitamin D and calcium levels. The screening and appropriate treatment of such deficiencies is an important part of managing hypothyroidism.

Selenium Selenium is an essential nutrient for supporting healthy thyroid metabolism, and studies have shown that it can help reduce Hashimoto's antibodies.

Zinc Zinc plays an important role in supporting thyroid and immune function. A zinc deficiency can compromise immune function, whereas adequate amounts of zinc can help increase the available form of the active thyroid hormone.

Also worth mentioning are cruciferous vegetables like broccoli, cauliflower, cabbage, bok choy, and Brussels sprouts. These vegetables were once restricted for those with thyroid conditions, but recent scientific literature does not support this recommendation, and the health benefits of this food group are far too substantial to ignore. Though it's not recommended to consume a large amount of raw cruciferous vegetables, a diet that includes a wide range of fruits and vegetables, including plenty of cooked cruciferous options, is most beneficial.

When to Reintroduce Foods

As mentioned earlier, the goal of the AIP is not to restrict all food groups indefinitely. In fact, it's not recommended to continue the elimination phase of the protocol beyond 90 days without the supervision of a medical professional. The majority of people who follow the AIP strictly for 60 to 90 days experience drastic results in the form of greatly reduced symptoms of their autoimmune condition. If symptom reduction is not seen during the elimination period, you'll want to follow up with your health care provider to ensure that no underlying problem needs to be addressed beyond dietary interventions.

Most people will experience some symptom relief within 30 to 60 days of starting the elimination phase of the protocol.

Once you feel well enough to begin the reintroduction phase, foods must be reintroduced in a specific order. The reintroduction strategy is based on each food's nutrient density and likelihood to cause an inflammatory response. For a more detailed guide to implementing the reintroduction phase, see "How to Reintroduce Foods" on page 179. This resource includes a symptom tracker to help you monitor your food reintroduction schedule and responses to it.

EASY, NUTRIENT-DENSE RECIPES

How do you make simple, healthy recipes that taste good *and* adhere to a strict protocol like the AIP? You combine the nutritional expertise of a registered dietitian with the culinary expertise of a chef.

When I explained to my chef husband what nightshades are and why he can't use them, he showed me what roulade, chimichurri, and agrodolce sauce are and how delicious they can be.

From late-night recipe planning to large dinners during which friends and family taste-tested our creations, we discovered the joy of working together in a professional capacity.

We got frustrated with recipes that just didn't work without the traditional ingredients we are used to, and we celebrated small wins when something turned out way better than expected (like the AIP-Friendly Fried Chicken, page 108). I learned how different cooking techniques could drastically change and improve the flavor of a dish, and he learned that coconut liquid aminos makes a pretty acceptable soy sauce substitute. In the end, we were able to combine flavor and nutrition to create the 105 easy, tasty, nutrient-dense dishes contained in this book.

The Hashimoto's AIP Cookbook takes away the need to scour the Internet for your favorite "AIP-approved" breakfasts, lunches, dinners, and snacks and puts them all in one place, along with some new favorites. Each recipe contains a delicious combination of anti-inflammatory, nutrient-rich ingredients that are free of the common inflammatory triggers that exacerbate symptoms. If you are living with Hashimoto's and are ready to follow the AIP, heal your gut, and put your symptoms to rest, simply pick a few recipes from chapters 3 through 9 of this book and get started on your journey to a better life!

If you are reading this book, you're probably already experiencing the oftentimes overwhelming symptoms of Hashimoto's, such as fatigue and brain fog. These symptoms make it difficult even to think about learning a detailed dietary protocol, much less implementing it. That's why the recipes in this book have been designed with convenience in mind. You'll notice that I've labeled each dish by its convenience attributes: 5-Ingredient, 30-Minute, Make-Ahead, or One-Pot/Pan/Bowl.

More than anything, the recipes in this book are designed to be high in flavor and satisfaction in order to make this new way of eating as pleasurable and stress-free as possible. Your family members will be able to enjoy many of the recipes in this book, eliminating the need to cook separate meals. Let's face it, food is more than a source of nourishment; it is also a source of pleasure and social connection. It's important to keep both alive and well to preserve your mental and emotional health while you work toward reclaiming your physical health. It is our hope that you will enjoy these recipes with family and friends and never feel deprived or unsatisfied.

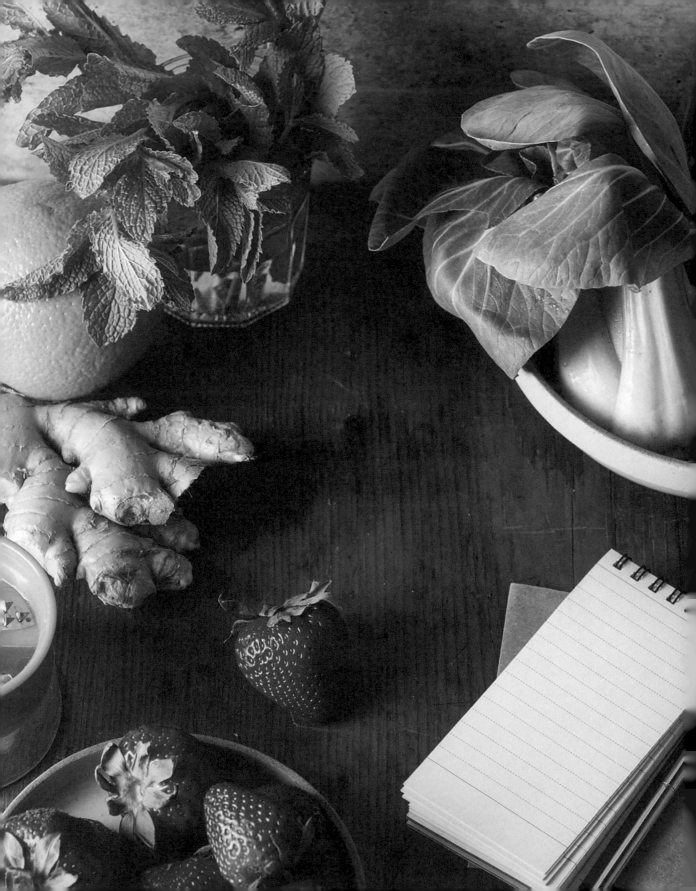

2 *Putting the AIP into Practice*

As a practitioner who walks clients through elimination diets, I can guess that you may be feeling overwhelmed at this point. I understand, and I want to invite you to take a deep breath and give a sigh of relief, because this chapter is going to take away your fear and replace that feeling with empowerment—and maybe even a little excitement. In the pages that follow, you will learn everything you need to know about adapting to the autoimmune protocol (AIP) in a sustainable, approachable way so you can enjoy the process, rather than stress over the unknown.

DIETARY RULES AND GUIDELINES

It may seem like there are a lot of rules, off-limit foods, and factors to consider when putting the AIP into practice. In the context of real life, there are many factors to consider before starting the protocol. Fortunately, a lot of the guidelines are easy to understand and even easier to implement. The purpose of this protocol is to eliminate inflammatory triggers from your diet and overall lifestyle by embracing the traditional concepts of hunting, gathering, and eating. By taking a step back in time to envision food fresh from the earth and meals made from scratch, you can easily turn away from the confusion of our current prepackaged society and embrace all the benefits of simplicity. Later in this chapter, we will explore more deeply the foods you can and cannot eat while on the protocol, but first we'll cover additional dietary considerations, such as the importance of quality, quantity, and variation.

Quality

The quality of the food you consume will play an important role in the implementation and effectiveness of the AIP. Although it is not always possible or necessary to buy all your produce organic, all your meat from a local butcher, or all your ingredients from a health food store, it is important to keep quality in mind. If your budget allows, purchase organic fruits and vegetables while in the elimination phase of the protocol. Many pesticides and other chemicals that are used in conventional farming can make their way from your food into your body, which is counterproductive when you're trying to give your body time to heal.

Certain pesticides and other chemicals are permitted in organic farming, so no matter which type of produce you choose to buy, be sure to wash it well to remove any residue. Because the benefits of eating conventional produce far outweigh the risks, it is better to eat produce from a conventional source than to eat no fresh produce.

When it comes to meat, keep in mind that the nutritional quality and health benefits of organic, grass-fed, free-range animal products are typically greater than those of traditionally farmed animal products. Consider visiting your local farm or butcher to find quality meat products obtained from humanely raised, healthy animals.

Quantity

As a dietitian, I try not to call the AIP a "diet" for fear that people may expect it to be a means of achieving weight loss. The AIP is not, and should not, be used as a fad diet or weight-loss tool, and counting or restricting calories on this protocol is not recommended. Healing cannot be achieved if adequate amounts of calories and nutrients are not consumed. While following the AIP, you should enjoy foods in reasonable amounts until you are full, and you should not leave the table feeling hungry or unsatisfied.

Variation

It may seem as if there are very few food options during the elimination phase of the protocol. In reality, many beneficial fruits and vegetables can add variation and satisfaction to your daily diet during the phase. It is important to explore a wide variety of foods and to not limit yourself to a few items. A variety of foods equals a variety of nutrients, which is necessary to achieve full healing and resolution of symptoms.

WHAT TO EAT (OR NOT EAT)

Sorting through what you can and cannot eat is one of the most overwhelming steps in this process. I want to make it as easy and enjoyable as possible to navigate your new (and temporary) dietary restrictions. Living by this simple set of rules will help guide you on your AIP journey and beyond:

1. *Load up on and eat meals filled with approved anti-inflammatory foods (see complete list, page 20)*
2. *Avoid processed and packaged foods*
3. *Avoid trans fats*
4. *Avoid added sugar*
5. *Avoid artificial sweeteners*

Rest easy knowing that every delicious recipe in this book is fully AIP-compliant, making your mealtime decisions quick and easy.

The AIP should not be approached with dread or hesitation, but instead with a spirit of positivity and excitement about healing. I expect that you are on your way to feeling better than you have in a long time. By first focusing on the foods you *can* enjoy freely, you'll avoid feeling overwhelmed and asking the dreaded question, "What is there left to eat?" I encourage you to focus on and embrace those AIP-compliant foods that you already love and enjoy, and to build your personalized diet on the basis of those foods. Your mind-set and satisfaction level will greatly affect your ability to stay the course and ultimately see results from the protocol.

Foods to Enjoy Freely

You are encouraged to enjoy meals filled with the following anti-inflammatory foods, which have antioxidants, omega-3 fatty acids, and plant-based dietary fiber, or some combination thereof. These foods are generally recognized as "safe" foods, but keep in mind your own personal sensitivities. In addition, choose organic produce whenever possible to avoid potential chemical sensitivities. Enjoy these foods without restriction:

Meats Organic, humanely raised, pastured chicken, turkey, duck, beef, pork, lamb, and venison

Wild-caught seafood Salmon, cod, halibut, trout, haddock, shrimp, lobster, clams, and mussels

Non-nightshade vegetables All vegetables except tomatoes, bell and hot peppers, eggplant, and white potatoes

High-quality oils Avocado oil, coconut oil, and extra-virgin olive oil

Healthy fats Avocado, coconut products, and bone broth

Fresh and dried herbs Parsley, thyme, basil, tarragon, rosemary, chives, chervil, marjoram, oregano, fennel, sage, lavender, mint, cilantro, and dill

Dairy-free fermented foods Kombucha, kefir, sauerkraut, kimchi, and vinegar

Beverages Herbal tea and homemade bone or vegetable broth

Condiments and pantry staples Nutritional yeast, collagen peptides, coconut liquid aminos, and root-based products like cassava flour and horseradish

Salt Talk to your health care provider about the quantity and type of salt you are using; different types of salt (iodized salt, sea salt, and so on) can have different minerals and thus different health implications.

Foods to Eat in Moderation

Though it is important to eat adequate amounts of calories and a wide variety of foods during the protocol, some foods should be consumed in moderation to minimize potential disruptions to blood sugar levels or other hormonal processes. The following foods provide beneficial nutrients, vitamins, minerals, phytonutrients, and antioxidants that are critical to the healing process, but they also contain sugar. Enjoy these foods in moderation:

Fresh fruit All types (2 to 3 servings per day—more for especially beneficial fibrous fruits like raspberries, blackberries, and strawberries)

Starchy vegetables Sweet potatoes, yams, squash, turnips, parsnips, and rutabagas (1 to 2 servings per day)

Dried fruit (¼ cup per day)

Natural sweeteners Pure maple syrup, raw honey, and coconut sugar

Foods to Restrict or Avoid

During the elimination phase of the protocol, strictly avoid the foods and food groups that can spark an inflammatory response in the body. Not every individual will be sensitive to all of the items listed here, but the protocol works by removing them for up to 90 days, thereby making the full protocol more likely to alleviate your unwanted symptoms, heal your gut, and put your autoimmune disease into remission. Eliminate these foods and food groups:

- ***Eggs***

- ***Dairy*** Milk from cows, sheep, goats, or any mammal, and any other food products derived from milk (butter, cheese, yogurt, ice cream, and whey protein)

- ***Grains*** Both gluten- and non-gluten-containing grains, including wheat, barley, rye, quinoa, rice, corn, oatmeal, millet, buckwheat, kamut, spelt, teff, amaranth, and sorghum

- ***Legumes*** Beans, peas, peanuts, soy in all forms (tofu, soy milk, edamame), and pod-based legumes (such as snap peas and green beans)

- ***Nightshade vegetables*** Tomatoes, peppers, eggplants, and white potatoes

- ***Nightshade-derived spices*** Dried chile flakes (such as red pepper flakes), capsicum, cayenne pepper, chili powder, curry, paprika, ancho, adobo

- ***Nuts*** All nuts, including almonds, walnuts, peanuts, nut butters like almond or cashew butter, and oils like walnut oil or sesame oil

- ***Seeds*** All seeds, including chia, flax, sunflower, pumpkin, hemp, and sesame

A Note on Spices

Determining which spices are allowed on the autoimmune protocol can be very confusing and even frustrating, so here is a guideline developed by Dr. Sarah Ballantyne to simplify your decision-making process. You can get more information in the resources section (page 184).

Safe spices Spices derived from the leaves, flowers, roots, and bark of a plant

Mild caution spices Spices derived from fruits and berries

Moderate caution spices Spices derived from seeds

High caution spices Spices derived from nightshades

- *Seed-derived spices* Black pepper, cumin seed, coriander seed, dill seed, fennel seed, fenugreek, mustard seed, celery seed, annatto seed, and anise seed

- *Vegetable oils* Soybean, corn, cottonseed, peanut, sunflower, safflower, canola, and palm oils

- *Artificial or processed meat products* Cured bacon, hot dogs, premade sausage, bologna, jerky, and deli meats

- *Artificial or refined sugar or sweeteners* White sugar, sucrose, high-fructose corn syrup, barley malt, dextrose, maltose, rice syrup, aspartame, saccharin, sucralose, acesulfame potassium, sorbitol, xylitol, monk fruit, and stevia

- *Anything artificial* Food additives, preservatives, and food dyes

- *Trans fats* Margarine, shortening, baked goods, packaged foods, and fast food

- *Alcohol, soda, and sugar-sweetened beverages*

Foods to Enjoy and Avoid

FOODS TO ENJOY	FOODS TO AVOID
Humanely raised, pastured meats (preferably organic): beef, bison, buffalo, chicken, duck, elk, lamb, mutton, pheasant, pork, quail, rabbit, turkey, venison, wild boar	**Artificial or processed meat products:** bologna, cured bacon, deli meats, hot dogs, jerky, premade sausage
Fresh fruit: apples, apricots, avocados, bananas, berries, cherries, cranberries, currants, dates, figs, grapes, grapefruit, kiwifruit, lemons, limes, mangos, mandarins, melons, nectarines, oranges, papayas, peaches, pears, plums, pineapple, plantains, pomegranates, pumpkins, rhubarb, tangerines	**Eggs and dairy products:** animal milk (from cows, sheep, goats, camels, or any other mammal), butter, cheese, ice cream, whey protein, yogurt
	Grains: amaranth, barley, buckwheat, corn, kamut, millet, oatmeal, quinoa, rice, rye, sorghum, spelt, teff, wheat
Dairy-free fermented foods: kombucha, kefir, apple cider vinegar, white wine vinegar, coconut vinegar, balsamic vinegar	**Legumes:** beans, peanuts, peas, soy in all forms (including tofu, soy milk, and edamame)
Wild-caught seafood: anchovies, catfish, clams, cod, crab, crawfish, haddock, halibut, herring, lobster, mahi-mahi, mussels, octopus, oysters, prawns, salmon, sardines, scallops, shrimp, snapper, tilapia, trout	**Mercury-contaminated seafood:** bluefish, grouper, mackerel, marlin, orange roughy, shark, swordfish, tilefish, tuna
	Nightshades and nightshade-derived spices: adobo, ancho, ashwagandha, bell peppers, capsicum, cayenne pepper, chiles (fresh and dried), chili powder, curry, eggplant, goji berries, gooseberries, huckle-berries, paprika, pimientos, red pepper flakes, tomatillos, tomatoes, white potatoes

Foods to Enjoy and Avoid

FOODS TO ENJOY	FOODS TO AVOID
Non-nightshade vegetables: artichokes, asparagus, beets, broccoli, Brussels sprouts, cabbage, carrots, cauliflower, celery, cucumbers, dark green leafy vegetables (arugula, bok choy, Swiss chard, collard greens, mustard greens, kale, lettuce, spinach), endive, fennel, jicama, kohlrabi, leeks, mushrooms, okra, olives, onions, parsnips, radishes, rapini (broccoli rabe), rutabagas, scallions, summer squash (zucchini and yellow squash), turnips, winter squash (acorn, butternut, delicata, kabocha, spaghetti squash), yuca root	**Nuts:** almonds, nut butters (almond butter, peanut butter, cashew butter, etc.), oils (walnut, sesame, peanut, etc.), peanuts, walnuts
High-quality oils: avocado, coconut, extra-virgin olive	**Seeds and seed-derived spices:** anise seeds, annatto seeds, celery seeds, chia, coriander seeds, cumin seeds, dill seeds, fennel seeds, fenugreek seeds, flaxseed, hemp seeds, mustard seeds, pepper and peppercorns (black, white, pink), pumpkin seeds, sesame seeds, sunflower seeds
Healthy fats: animal fat (lard and tallow from pastured, grass-fed animals), avocado, bone broth, coconut products	**Vegetable oils:** canola, corn, cotton-seed, palm, peanut, soybean, safflower, sunflower
Fresh or dried herbs and spices: basil, bay leaf, chervil, chives, cilantro, cinnamon, dill, fennel, ginger, lavender, marjoram, mint, oregano, parsley, peppermint, rosemary, saffron, sage, tarragon, thyme, turmeric	**Artificial or refined sugar or sweeteners**
Sweeteners (in moderation): coconut sugar, honey (raw), maple syrup (pure)	**Anything artificial**
	Trans fats

Please remember that you are not to restrict all of these foods for longer than 60 to 90 days without medical supervision. Many of these foods and food groups contain healthy nutrients and beneficial properties that will enhance your overall diet quality during and after the reintroduction phase.

Additionally, remember that the inflammatory process is unique to each individual. A dietary trigger for one person may not be a trigger for another. The goal here is to create a personalized diet reflecting your unique needs and offering the greatest variety of foods.

SETTING YOURSELF UP FOR SUCCESS

To find success with the autoimmune protocol, you'll need to learn how to fall in love with cooking meals from scratch. Good health and good nutrition start with the preparation of wholesome, home-cooked meals. Cooking at home allows you to have complete control over ingredients, which is good for your health and your peace of mind. A well-stocked and thoughtfully organized kitchen can help make implementing the protocol easy, enjoyable, and stress-free. Let's start with a meal plan.

Beverages and Drinks

When following any elimination diet, you can easily forget about beverages. Just like foods, some drinks provide important nutrients and health benefits, and others aggravate or ignite inflammation. Drink enough nutritious beverages to stay hydrated. Adequate hydration facilitates healing and is vital to supporting the body's natural detox pathways.

Drinks to Enjoy

- Bone broth
- Coconut milk without additives
- Filtered water—can be enhanced with AIP-approved ingredients like lemon, mint, berries, cucumber, or ginger
- Freshly juiced fruits or vegetables
- Herbal tea—hot or iced
- Kombucha
- Smoothies made from AIP-approved ingredients

Drinks to Avoid

- Alcohol
- Artificially sweetened beverages
- Caffeinated beverages
- Coffee—decaf and regular
- Energy drinks
- Fruit juice from concentrate
- Milk—dairy and nut/seed-based
- Sugar-sweetened beverages
- Soda—diet and regular

Sample Two-Week Meal Plan

Meal Prep Ahead of Time: Creamy Coconut Milk Yogurt (page 177), Sweet Potato Breakfast Skillet (page 43), Slow Cooker Shredded Chicken (page 107), From-Scratch Cauliflower Rice (page 60), Garlic Mashed Rutabagas (page 69), AIP-Friendly Flatbread (page 176), Lemon Parsnip Hummus (page 49), Baked Coconut Macaroon Bites (page 155)

	Breakfast	Lunch	Dinner	Snack
DAY 1	Raspberry Cinnamon Yogurt Bowl (page 39)	Chilled Mango Salmon Salad Wraps (page 72)	Sunday Supper Pot Roast (page 132) with Garlic Mashed Rutabagas (page 69)	AIP-Friendly Flatbread (page 176), vegetables, Lemon Parsnip Hummus (page 49)
DAY 2	Sweet Potato Breakfast Skillet (page 43)	Leftover Sunday Supper Pot Roast (page 132) with Garlic Mashed Rutabagas (page 69)	Greek Salmon en Papillote (page 76) with From-Scratch Cauliflower Rice (page 60)	Baked Coconut Macaroon Bites (page 155)
DAY 3	Anti-Inflammatory Matcha Latte (page 34)	Grape Chicken Salad Wraps (page 100)	Chicken Egg Roll in a Bowl (page 105)	AIP-Friendly Flatbread (page 176), vegetables, Lemon Parsnip Hummus (page 49)
DAY 4	Mango Turmeric Lassi (page 35)	Chilled Mango Salmon Salad Wraps (page 72)	Mediterranean Chicken Pizzas (page 102) with Chimichurri Baked Chicken Wings (page 104)	Honey Cinnamon Fruit Salad (page 147)
DAY 5	Raspberry Cinnamon Yogurt Bowl (page 39)	Leftover Chicken Egg Roll in a Bowl (page 105) with From-Scratch Cauliflower Rice (page 60)	Dutch Oven Pork with Apples and Fennel (page 118) with Garlic Mashed Rutabagas (page 69)	Two-Ingredient Grape Gelatin (page 146)
DAY 6	Triple Berry Antioxidant Smoothie (page 37)	Grape Chicken Salad Wraps (page 100)	Lemon Spinach Turkey Soup (page 94) with AIP-Friendly Flatbread (page 176)	Baked Coconut Macaroon Bites (page 155)
DAY 7	Sweet Potato Breakfast Skillet (page 43)	Leftover Dutch Oven Pork with Apples and Fennel (page 118) with leftover From-Scratch Cauliflower Rice (page 60) or Garlic Mashed Rutabagas (page 69)	Portobello Mushroom Beef Burgers (page 133) with Baked Rutabaga French Fries (page 57)	Honey Cinnamon Fruit Salad (page 147)

Meal Prep Ahead of Time: Creamy Coconut Milk Yogurt (page 177), Breakfast Sausage and Cauli-Hash (page 44), Cinnamon Baked Sweet Potato Chips (page 56), Grain-Free Tortillas (page 174), Apricot Date Energy Bites (page 142), Strawberry Fruit Tart (page 152)

	Breakfast	Lunch	Dinner	Snack
DAY 8	Anti-Inflammatory Matcha Latte (page 34)	Cranberry Salmon Spinach Salad (page 73)	Bok Choy Pork Stir-Fry (page 120)	Strawberry Fruit Tart (page 152)
DAY 9	Wild Blueberry Coconut Milk Yogurt (page 38)	Leftover Bok Choy Pork Stir-Fry (page 120)	Mexican Cod Fish Tacos (page 80) with Creamy Pineapple Coleslaw (page 51) in Grain-Free Tortillas (page 174)	Apricot Date Energy Bites (page 142)
DAY 10	Breakfast Sausage and Cauli-Hash (page 44)	Lemon Basil Chicken Sliders (page 101) with Cinnamon Baked Sweet Potato Chips (page 56)	Churrasco Skirt Steak with Chimichurri (page 126)	Tropical Mango Gelato (page 148)
DAY 11	Caramelized Plantain Porridge (page 41)	Leftover Churrasco Skirt Steak with Chimichurri (page 126) with Shredded Brussels Sprout Salad (page 55)	Mediterranean Lamb Meatballs (page 134) in Roasted Spaghetti Squash Bowls (page 66)	Strawberry Fruit Tart (page 152)
DAY 12	Bright Green Detox Smoothie (page 36)	Cranberry Salmon Spinach Salad (page 73)	One-Pot Shrimp Bisque (page 90)	Apricot Date Energy Bites (page 142)
DAY 13	Breakfast Sausage and Cauli-Hash (page 44)	Lemon Basil Chicken Sliders (page 101) with Cinnamon Baked Sweet Potato Chips (page 56)	One-Pot Whole Roasted Chicken (page 112) with Savory Pumpkin Gnocchi (page 58)	Tropical Mango Gelato (page 148)
DAY 14	Caramelized Plantain Porridge (page 41)	Leftover One-Pot Shrimp Bisque (page 90)	Mediterranean Chicken Pizzas (page 102) made with leftover One-Pot Whole Roasted Chicken (page 112)	Strawberry Fruit Tart (page 152)

Essential Kitchen Equipment

A clean and well-organized kitchen can set you up for success that will last long after the AIP has ended. The first step is to dedicate a small area in the kitchen to recipe preparation. It can be a section of countertop or your kitchen table. Next, secure a safe and reliable stove, oven, grill, or slow cooker, and make sure it is clean and in good working condition before starting to cook.

Finally, ensure that you have the right tools to help you make your recipes quickly and easily.

MUST-HAVE EQUIPMENT

Knives A good set of sharp knives is integral to cooking ease, success, and safety.

Cutting board A large, sturdy cutting board is best. Place a damp towel under it to keep the board from shifting.

Pots and pans A set of various-size pots and pans will allow you to cook all this book's recipes, even without a slow cooker, Instant Pot, or other cooking appliance.

Blender A high-powered blender will make prep for smoothies, soups, dressings, and other foods easy.

Digital instant-read thermometer Food safety is imperative to have a safe and enjoyable cooking experience. This book calls for using the thermometer often to ensure that all your dishes, especially meat, poultry, and seafood, are cooked to the proper temperature.

High-temperature rubber spatula This kitchen tool will allow you to easily mix your hot ingredients.

NICE-TO-HAVE EQUIPMENT

Food processor A food processor can chop, dice, and shred various foods quickly and easily.

Mandoline This cutting tool slices fruits and vegetables in a uniform shape and size. (Exercise extreme caution when using this very sharp tool.)

Spiralizer A spiralizer can quickly turn zucchini, yellow squash, carrots, beets, and sweet potatoes into vegetable "noodles"—helpful for a grain-free diet!

Immersion blender Although a traditional blender will do just fine, this tool can make soups and dressings even easier to create.

Pantry Essentials

Most of the recipes in this book require no more than 30 minutes. Many call for five or fewer ingredients, use one pot or pan, or can be made ahead of time. Furthermore, these recipes generally rely on familiar ingredients that you can easily find at your local grocery store. Though a few ingredients may be new to you, like collagen protein, cassava flour, or coconut cream, they can all be found in health food stores or online. To avoid multiple grocery shopping trips for this book's recipes, try to keep the following must-have items on hand:

Pantry Items

- Coconut liquid aminos
- Coconut products (full-fat coconut milk, light coconut milk, coconut cream, unsweetened coconut flakes, coconut butter)
- Grain and nut-free flours (cassava, coconut, tigernut)
- Nutritional yeast
- Oils (coconut, extra-virgin olive, avocado)
- Pure vanilla extract
- Raw honey, pure maple syrup, and coconut sugar
- Unflavored collagen peptides and gelatin
- Vinegars (apple cider, white, balsamic)

Spice Rack

- Dried basil
- Dried mint
- Dried oregano
- Dried parsley
- Dried thyme
- Garlic powder
- Ground ginger
- Ground turmeric
- Onion powder
- Sea salt (which can be used interchangeably with kosher salt)
- Table salt

Refrigerator Items

- Chicken, turkey, beef, and pork (organic, grass-fed, pastured if possible)

- Fresh fruits and vegetables (organic if possible)
- Homemade bone broth
- Probiotics to make yogurt

Freezer Items

- Chicken, turkey, beef, and pork (organic, grass-fed, pastured if possible)
- Fish and seafood like cod, halibut, and shrimp (wild-caught if possible)

- Frozen tropical fruits and berries
- Frozen vegetables like cauliflower and cauliflower rice
- Homemade bone broth

10 HANDY PERISHABLES

You may find yourself buying a few staple items week after week, so why not note these items and keep them available? These 10 items are frequently used in this book's recipes:

1. Garlic
2. Fresh gingerroot
3. Organic cuts of chicken
4. Organic cuts of beef
5. Sweet potatoes
6. Lemon juice
7. Mirepoix (celery, carrots, onion)
8. Cauliflower (whole head, florets, or riced)
9. Dark green leafy vegetables (spinach, kale)
10. Homemade bone broth (beef, pork, chicken, or even vegetable bone broth)

Note: If your time or energy is limited, purchase these items already prepared. For example, you can buy minced garlic rather than whole cloves and riced cauliflower instead of a whole cauliflower.

Effort-Saving Tips

One of the greatest challenges of sticking with any new diet is feeling confident enough to prepare the food for yourself. No matter how delicious the recipes are, if they're too hard to prepare, you'll never find the time to make or enjoy them. Rest assured that this book's recipes are easy to follow, enjoyable to prepare, and, of course, delicious to eat. Here are a few tips and shortcuts to make your at-home cooking experience easy:

BUY PRE-CUT FRUITS AND VEGETABLES

Grocery stores recognize the need for convenience, and so many offer pre-cut fruits and vegetables. Though these items tend to be more expensive than uncut items, they can be major time-savers in the kitchen. If possible, purchase pre-cut carrots, coleslaw mix, broccoli and cauliflower florets, vegetable noodles, diced rutabagas, and pre-cut sweet potato French fries. Always read package labels to ensure that no additional ingredients are included.

BUY FROZEN FRUITS AND VEGETABLES

Frozen fruits and vegetables are just as nutritious as fresh fruits and vegetables, because they are typically frozen at peak freshness, locking in important nutrients. Plus, frozen produce is often more affordable than fresh produce, and it comes already washed and cut, which reduces your time in the kitchen. Always read package labels to ensure that no additional ingredients are included.

COOK IN BULK AND UTILIZE MAKE-AHEAD RECIPES

If you know you're going to enjoy more than one recipe with cauliflower rice during the week, prepare the cauliflower rice in a double or triple batch. The same goes for meats such as chicken, pork, and beef. Double or triple the recipe as needed, and then freeze extra portions in individual serving sizes. This "cook once, eat twice" method of preparation reduces effort and gives you options to fall back on if your plans or health changes drastically, upsetting your cooking schedule.

USE STORE-BOUGHT OPTIONS

Not all prepackaged and store-bought items are created equal. A quick scan of the ingredients list can help you determine if a packaged food is right for you. Consider purchasing items like organic bone broth and kombucha made with a few safe, recognizable ingredients to make recipe preparation easy. You can also find pre-packaged staple items, like riced cauliflower, in the fresh or frozen section of the grocery store.

PLAN A DAY TO MEAL PREP

Many people don't have enough time or energy to prepare healthy meals every day, so it can be very helpful to designate one day of the week for meal planning and prepping. You don't have to dedicate the entire day to this effort—just set aside a few hours to prepare a few staple items.

HEALTHY LIFESTYLE CHANGES

This book focuses on the dietary changes to help reduce and reverse symptoms of Hashimoto's disease. That said, the proper management of Hashimoto's disease requires a complete holistic lifestyle approach, which, in addition to dietary modifications, involves taking medications as prescribed by your doctor, working with your multidisciplinary health care team to develop an appropriate supplement regimen, implementing an enjoyable exercise routine, and caring for your mental and emotional health, especially as it relates to stress management.

To ensure that your dietary efforts are effective, take other lifestyle factors into consideration. Big moves like quitting smoking and abstaining from alcohol and recreational drugs are imperative for the success of the autoimmune protocol. Over-the-counter (OTC) and prescription medications should be considered, too. OTC medications like nonsteroidal anti-inflammatory drugs can damage the gut lining and may sabotage your efforts, and some prescription medications are manufactured with off-limits ingredients like corn or soy. Do your research so you know exactly what you are putting in your body, and always talk to your physician before making any medication changes.

Many people find that what they put *on* their bodies also affects their health and recovery. Your skin is your body's largest organ, and it, too, can absorb toxic chemicals from everyday household items such as shampoo, lotion, and cleaning products. Choose these items wisely, and look into natural products.

Finally, good sleep hygiene is critical to the resumption of good health, especially when symptoms like fatigue and brain fog are involved. Developing a consistent bedtime routine will help you adopt the good sleep habits needed to support your body as you heal. Try to go to sleep at the same time every night, minimize distractions in the bedroom, and focus on sleep-promoting activities like turning off electronics, using essential oils, or meditating.

By putting all of these important lifestyle changes into place before or while implementing the AIP, you will set yourself up for success during and after the diet.

ABOUT THE RECIPES

If you are closing out this chapter feeling overwhelmed in any way, I want to assure you that the hard work was already done for you. All the recipes in this book have been chef-created and dietitian-approved for the best combination of flavor and nutrition. Additionally, every single recipe strictly follows the AIP guidelines, taking the guesswork out of cooking.

Of course, you still need to prepare the recipes, which can be especially difficult if you are not feeling well or are experiencing debilitating symptoms as a result of your autoimmune condition. Spending hours on end in the kitchen is neither feasible nor realistic, so every recipe in this book comes with at least one of the following labels: 5-Ingredient, 30-Minute, Make-Ahead, or One-Pot/Pan/Bowl. These labels will assist you in planning or prepping your weekly meals and will allow you to create a meal plan that is convenient as well as health-supportive.

Recipe Labels Decoded

5-Ingredient The recipe calls for no more than five ingredients, not including salt, pepper, and olive oil, making it simple to prepare.

30-Minute The entire recipe can be made from start to finish, prep to plate, in no more than 30 minutes.

Make-Ahead The recipe can be made ahead of time and stored in the pantry, refrigerator, or freezer for future use.

One-Pot/Pan/Bowl The entire recipe can be made in a single pot, pan, bowl, or other container/appliance, alleviating the stress of having multiple dishes to clean up.

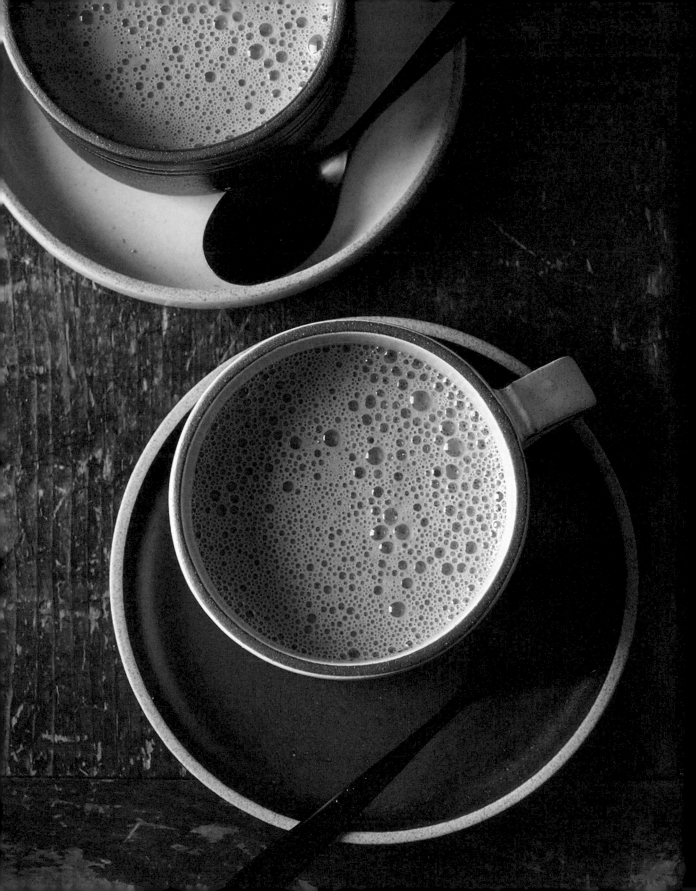

3 Smoothies and Breakfasts

Anti-Inflammatory Matcha Latte

Matcha is a Japanese tea that is made of a finely ground powder of green tea leaves specially cultivated for the creation of matcha tea. This healing, frothy drink has a smooth, earthy flavor and is typically made by whisking the green tea powder into boiling water. Because you are consuming the whole tea leaves, you get more of the powerful nutritional benefits of green tea. Polyphenols, the antioxidants most present in matcha, have been shown to boost metabolism and may even help protect against heart disease and cancer. **MAKES 2 SERVINGS**

¼ cup filtered water

2 teaspoons pure matcha powder

2 cups light coconut milk

1 tablespoon coconut sugar

½ teaspoon ground ginger

½ teaspoon pure vanilla extract

2 tablespoons unflavored collagen peptides (optional)

30-MINUTE ONE-POT

Cook time: 10 minutes

Ingredient Tip: Though the collagen peptides are optional in this recipe, I strongly recommend that you add them whenever you can for their nutritional value. Each tablespoon of collagen peptides provides 10 grams of high-quality protein that can help the gut heal and keep you full and satisfied after your morning meal.

1. In a medium saucepan over medium-high heat, bring the water to a boil. Turn off the heat, and whisk in the matcha powder to form a paste.

2. Return the heat to low and stir in the coconut milk, coconut sugar, and ginger. Cook on low, stirring occasionally, for 5 minutes, or until just boiling.

3. Just before serving, stir in the vanilla extract and collagen peptides (if using).

Per Serving (1 cup): Calories: 164; Total Fat: 12g; Saturated Fat: 11g; Sodium: 60mg; Carbohydrates: 16g; Fiber: 1g; Protein: 4g

Mango Turmeric Lassi

A lassi is a traditional Indian drink that combines yogurt, water, spices, and sometimes fruit. The main healing agent in this recipe is turmeric, a versatile spice shown to support a healthy inflammatory response in the body. Though turmeric is traditionally paired with black pepper to maximize absorption, this drink instead capitalizes on a serving of fruit and vegetables for a wholesome, nutritious morning treat. **MAKES 2 SERVINGS**

1 cup diced
frozen mango

1 cup sliced
frozen carrots

1 cup Creamy
Coconut Milk Yogurt
(page 177)

1 cup filtered water

1 tablespoon pure
maple syrup

½ teaspoon ground
turmeric

2 tablespoons
unflavored collagen
peptides (optional)

**30-MINUTE
ONE-BOWL**

Prep time: 5 minutes

1. To a blender, add the mango, carrots, coconut milk yogurt, water, maple syrup, turmeric, and collagen peptides (if using).

2. Blend on high for 2 minutes, or until completely smooth.

Per Serving (1 cup): Calories: 341; Total Fat: 24g; Saturated Fat: 21g; Sodium: 55mg; Carbohydrates: 36g; Fiber: 6g; Protein: 1g

Ingredient Tip: Frozen fruits and vegetables are just as nutritious as fresh, as long as there are no other added ingredients. Purchasing frozen fruit helps to cut down on prep time, can save you money, and makes for a cold, creamy consistency that's perfect for this drink.

Ingredient Tip: Though the collagen peptides are optional in this recipe, I strongly recommend that you add them whenever you can for their nutritional value. Each tablespoon of collagen peptides provides 10 grams of high-quality protein that can help the gut heal and keep you full and satisfied after your morning meal.

Bright Green Detox Smoothie

This smoothie is not only packed with spinach, which contains vitamins C and K, folic acid, iron, and calcium, but it also contains celery stalks and cucumber, both shown to aid the body in its natural detox processes. Celery has powerful anti-inflammatory effects and may help naturally manage high blood pressure and promote heart health. Not limited to just breakfast, smoothies are a great way to get in additional servings of fruits and vegetables throughout the day.

MAKES 2 SERVINGS

2 celery stalks, diced

1 avocado, pitted and scooped

1 cup baby spinach, packed

1 green apple, cored and diced

1 small cucumber, diced

½-inch piece peeled fresh gingerroot

1 cup ice cubes

1 cup freshly squeezed orange juice or filtered water

2 tablespoons unflavored collagen peptides (optional)

30-MINUTE
ONE-BOWL

Prep time: 5 minutes

1. To a blender, add the celery, avocado, spinach, apple, cucumber, ginger, ice, orange juice, and collagen peptides (if using).

2. Blend on high for 2 minutes, or until completely smooth.

Per Serving (1 cup): Calories: 291; Total Fat: 14g; Saturated Fat: 2g; Sodium: 38mg; Carbohydrates: 43g; Fiber: 10g; Protein: 5g

Substitution Tip: Green smoothies are so versatile, and the ingredients can be interchanged and still taste yummy. If you are struggling with the taste of a green smoothie, try adding in a frozen banana. This will make the recipe creamier and sweeter.

Ingredient Tip: Though the collagen peptides are optional in this recipe, I strongly recommend that you add them whenever you can for their nutritional value. Each tablespoon of collagen peptides provides 10 grams of high-quality protein that can help the gut heal and keep you full and satisfied after your morning meal.

Triple Berry Antioxidant Smoothie

Smoothies are a delicious way to enjoy fruits and veggies first thing in the morning. A main ingredient in this smoothie is cauliflower, which lends a mellow flavor and a smooth and creamy texture. Cauliflower, a good source of antioxidants, also contains important nutrients like vitamins C, K, and B$_6$, as well as potassium and magnesium. The berries are a powerful source of antioxidants that can help fight free radicals in the body. **MAKES 2 SERVINGS**

2 small cooked beets

1 cup frozen cauliflower florets

1 cup frozen strawberries

½ cup frozen blueberries

½ cup frozen raspberries

2 cups light coconut milk

1 teaspoon pure vanilla extract

1 teaspoon pure maple syrup

½ teaspoon ground cinnamon

2 tablespoons unflavored collagen peptides (optional)

30-MINUTE ONE-BOWL

Prep time: 5 minutes

1. To a blender, add the beets, cauliflower, berries, coconut milk, vanilla, maple syrup, cinnamon, and collagen peptides (if using).

2. Blend on high for 2 minutes, or until completely smooth.

Per Serving (1 cup): Calories: 318; Total Fat: 13g; Saturated Fat: 11g; Sodium: 153mg; Carbohydrates: 52g; Fiber: 9g; Protein: 6g

Substitution Tip: Feel free to use whatever frozen berries you have on hand. All berries are a good source of antioxidants and dietary fiber, which will help keep you fuller, longer.

Ingredient Tip: Though the collagen peptides are optional in this recipe, I strongly recommend that you add them whenever you can for their nutritional value. Each tablespoon of collagen peptides provides 10 grams of high-quality protein that can help the gut heal and keep you full and satisfied after your morning meal.

Wild Blueberry Coconut Milk Yogurt

Wild blueberries contain important dietary nutrients without adding a lot of extra calories. At just 80 calories per cup, these berries are loaded with antioxidants and pack a serious nutritional punch in every calorie. They are naturally low in fat and high in fiber (twice the amount of regular blueberries), and they have no added sugar, sodium, or refined starches. **MAKES 4 SERVINGS**

2 cups Creamy Coconut Milk Yogurt (page 177)

1 cup frozen wild blueberries, thawed

¼ cup unflavored collagen peptides

2 tablespoons pure maple syrup

2 tablespoons unsweetened shredded coconut flakes

5-INGREDIENT
30-MINUTE
MAKE-AHEAD
ONE-BOWL

Prep time: 5 minutes

1. In a large bowl, mix together the coconut milk yogurt, thawed blueberries, collagen peptides, maple syrup, and shredded coconut. Mix well.

2. Divide the coconut milk yogurt among 4 bowls for serving.

Per Serving (¾ cup): Calories: 332; Total Fat: 28g; Saturated Fat: 25g; Sodium: 26mg; Carbohydrates: 20g; Fiber: 4g; Protein: 3g

Substitution Tip: You can find wild blueberries in the freezer section of your local supermarket. Feel free to swap out the wild blueberries for any berry you enjoy, like raspberries or blackberries, for a different flavor profile.

Ingredient Tip: Studies have shown that collagen is an important nutrient to help heal leaky gut. You can find collagen peptides at your local health food store or online.

Make-Ahead Tip: To save time, make this recipe ahead of time and store it in individual grab-and-go containers for easy and nutritious breakfasts all week long. Refrigerate for up to 5 days.

Raspberry Cinnamon Yogurt Bowl

Many people find breakfast to be the most difficult meal while following the AIP because common breakfast staples like grains and eggs are restricted. Fortunately, coconut milk yogurt is easy to make at home, free of common additives and artificial ingredients, and completely versatile. This yogurt bowl is a blank canvas for many wonderful breakfast and snack variations. **MAKES 4 SERVINGS**

¼ cup unsweetened
   coconut flakes
2 cups Creamy
   Coconut Milk Yogurt
   (page 177)
¼ cup unflavored
   collagen peptides

2 tablespoons pure
   maple syrup
½ teaspoon pure
   vanilla extract
½ teaspoon ground
   cinnamon
2 cups fresh red
   raspberries

5-INGREDIENT
30-MINUTE
MAKE-AHEAD

Prep time: 5 minutes

Substitution Tip: Try diced pears or apples to add dietary fiber and nutrients.

Serving Tip: Enjoy the cinnamon coconut yogurt as is, or use it as a topping for sweet treats such as Slow Cooker Poached Pears (page 150) or as a filling for the Strawberry Fruit Tart (page 152).

Ingredient Tip: Studies have shown that collagen is an important nutrient to help heal leaky gut. You can find collagen peptides at your local health food store or online.

1. In a small skillet over medium-high heat, toast the coconut flakes for 60 to 90 seconds, stirring constantly, until golden brown. Set aside.

2. In a large bowl, mix together the coconut milk yogurt, collagen peptides, maple syrup, vanilla, and cinnamon. Mix well.

continued

3. Divide the mixture among 4 bowls.

4. Top each yogurt bowl with ½ cup fresh red raspberries and 1 tablespoon toasted coconut flakes.

   Make-Ahead Tip: Store individual servings in grab-and-go containers, such as Mason jars, for no-fuss breakfasts all week long. Refrigerate for up to 5 days.

Per Serving (½ cup yogurt, ½ cup fresh raspberries, 1 tablespoon coconut flakes): Calories: 318; Total Fat: 26g; Saturated Fat: 23g; Sodium: 25mg; Carbohydrates: 21g; Fiber: 7g; Protein: 3g

Caramelized Plantain Porridge

Plantains are dense and starchy, and they make the perfect thick and creamy grain-free base for porridge. Naturally vegan and gluten-free, this plant-based recipe relies on coconut milk and turmeric for its anti-inflammatory compounds and beautiful yellow color. **MAKES 4 SERVINGS**

1 tablespoon
    coconut oil
2 ripe plantains, diced
2 cups coconut milk
1 teaspoon pure
    vanilla extract
¼ teaspoon ground
    turmeric

¼ teaspoon
    ground ginger
1 tablespoon
    coconut sugar
¼ cup unflavored
    collagen peptides
    (optional)

**30-MINUTE
ONE-POT**

Prep time: 5 minutes
Cook time: 15 minutes

Recipe Tip: Use a combination of spices to make this dish your own. Cinnamon, grated fresh gingerroot, coconut flakes, and pure maple syrup all make excellent additions to this dish.

Ingredient Tip: Studies have shown that collagen is an important nutrient to help heal leaky gut. You can find collagen peptides at your local health food store or online.

1. In a large skillet over medium heat, melt the coconut oil.

2. Once the oil is hot, add the plantains and cook for 5 minutes, stirring occasionally, allowing them to caramelize and turn golden brown.

3. Pour in the coconut milk and stir in the vanilla, turmeric, and ginger.

4. Bring the mixture to a boil, then reduce the heat to a simmer and cover with a tight-fitting lid. Simmer for 5 minutes.

5. Remove the lid and gently mash the plantains with a potato masher or large fork. Return the lid and simmer for another 5 minutes.

6. Remove the skillet from the heat and stir in the coconut sugar and collagen peptides (if using) just before serving.

Per Serving (¾ cup): Calories: 440; Total Fat: 32g; Saturated Fat: 28g; Sodium: 29mg; Carbohydrates: 39g; Fiber: 5g; Protein: 6g

Bacon Date Spinach Sauté

A hearty breakfast may seem like a thing of the past on the AIP, but this delicious recipe will have you feeling full and satisfied, without the eggs or toast. Uncured bacon is bacon that has not been cured with sodium nitrates. Though it's not an everyday ingredient, uncured bacon is a delicious addition to a breakfast-time meal, and it pairs well with the natural sweetness of the dates. **MAKES 4 SERVINGS**

12 ounces uncured
   bacon, diced
12 dates, pitted
   and diced
2 cups riced cauliflower

6 cups baby
   spinach, packed
1 teaspoon pure
   maple syrup
½ teaspoon salt

5-INGREDIENT
30-MINUTE
ONE-POT

Prep time: 10 minutes
Cook time: 20 minutes

1. Place the diced bacon in a cold skillet on the stovetop. Turn the heat to medium-low and allow the bacon to cook for 7 minutes, stirring occasionally, until it begins to turn slightly golden brown.

2. Turn off the heat and carefully drain approximately three-quarters of the fat from the pan. Save or discard the fat.

3. Return the pan to the stove over medium heat, and add the dates and cauliflower rice. Cook for 2 minutes, stirring frequently.

4. Add the packed spinach by the handful, letting it wilt before you add more to the pan. Stir until all the spinach is wilted, about 3 minutes.

5. Turn off the heat; stir in the maple syrup and salt before serving.

Ingredient Tip: You can use any type of dark leafy green in place of the spinach. Switch things up and try kale, Swiss chard, collard greens, or even turnip greens.

Serving Tip: For a big breakfast, pair this recipe with Hasselback Baked Sweet Potatoes (page 67).

Per Serving (¼ prepared recipe): Calories: 452; Total Fat: 34g; Saturated Fat: 11g; Sodium: 905mg; Carbohydrates: 25g; Fiber: 4g; Protein: 14g

Sweet Potato Breakfast Skillet

This one-pot breakfast will keep you full all morning long. Sweet potatoes are rich in the antioxidant beta-carotene and in minerals like iron, calcium, and selenium. They also provide complex carbohydrates and are a rich source of dietary fiber. Paired with dried cranberries, which add a hint of sweetness, this breakfast is the perfect combination of sweet and savory. **MAKES 4 SERVINGS**

1 tablespoon
   coconut oil
4 sweet potatoes,
   peeled and
   finely diced
¼ teaspoon salt
1 pound ground pork

1 tablespoon AIP Spice
   Blend (page 160)
½ cup unsweetened
   dried cranberries
1 teaspoon chopped
   fresh sage
¼ cup filtered water

**30-MINUTE
ONE-POT**

Prep time: 10 minutes
Cook time: 20 minutes

Ingredient Tip: Use any ground meat you desire in this recipe: ground beef, lamb, chicken, pork, or turkey.

Substitution Tip: You can substitute unsweetened dried cherries or raisins for the dried cranberries. If you don't have fresh sage, feel free to substitute ¼ teaspoon dried sage.

1. In a large skillet over medium-high heat, melt the coconut oil.

2. When the oil is hot, add the sweet potatoes and salt. Allow to cook for 10 minutes, stirring occasionally to prevent sticking.

3. Push the sweet potatoes to the edges of the skillet. Add the ground meat to the middle of the skillet and cook for 5 minutes, stirring occasionally.

4. When the pork is cooked through and there is no pink left, stir in the spice blend, dried cranberries, and sage. Stir well and cook for 2 additional minutes.

5. Reduce the heat to low, add the water, and cook for 1 additional minute.

Per Serving (¼ prepared recipe): Calories: 379; Total Fat: 20g; Saturated Fat: 9g; Sodium: 299mg; Carbohydrates: 28g; Fiber: 5g; Protein: 22g

Breakfast Sausage and Cauli-Hash

Hash is a classic dish made with diced or chopped meat, potatoes, and spices that are mixed and cooked together. Traditional premade breakfast sausage may contain ingredients that are not allowed on the AIP. This sausage—made with dried herbs and ground pork, a high-quality source of protein and many important nutrients like iron and B vitamins—will fit perfectly in your AIP routine.

MAKES 4 SERVINGS

1 pound ground pork
1 tablespoon AIP Spice Blend (page 160)
1 tablespoon coconut sugar
½ teaspoon salt
2 tablespoons coconut oil
4 cups riced cauliflower
¾ cup Homemade Vegetable Bone Broth (page 162)
¼ cup coconut cream

30-MINUTE
Prep time: 10 minutes
Cook time: 20 minutes

Cooking Tip: You can prepare and cook the sausage patties separately from the rest of the dish to use with other breakfast meals.

1. In a large bowl, mix together the pork, spice blend, coconut sugar, and salt with your hands until well incorporated.

2. Shape the sausage into 1-inch balls and then press them flat to create eight 2-inch-wide patties.

3. In a cast-iron skillet over medium-high heat, melt the coconut oil.

4. When the oil is hot, add the sausage patties one at a time, being careful to avoid oil splatters.

5. Cook for 5 minutes, or until the edges begin to brown, then flip and cook the patties for another 5 minutes, or until they reach an internal temperature of 145°F. Remove the patties from the pan and place them on a paper towel to wick away excess oil.

6. Add the riced cauliflower and broth to the skillet and cook for 5 minutes, stirring occasionally.

7. Reduce the heat to low and stir in the coconut cream. Push the cauli-hash to the edges of the pan.

8. Return the sausage patties to the pan to warm, and serve them over the cauli-hash.

Per Serving (2 sausage patties, ½ cup cauli-hash): Calories: 418; Total Fat: 33g; Saturated Fat: 20g; Sodium: 401mg; Carbohydrates: 9g; Fiber: 3g; Protein: 23g

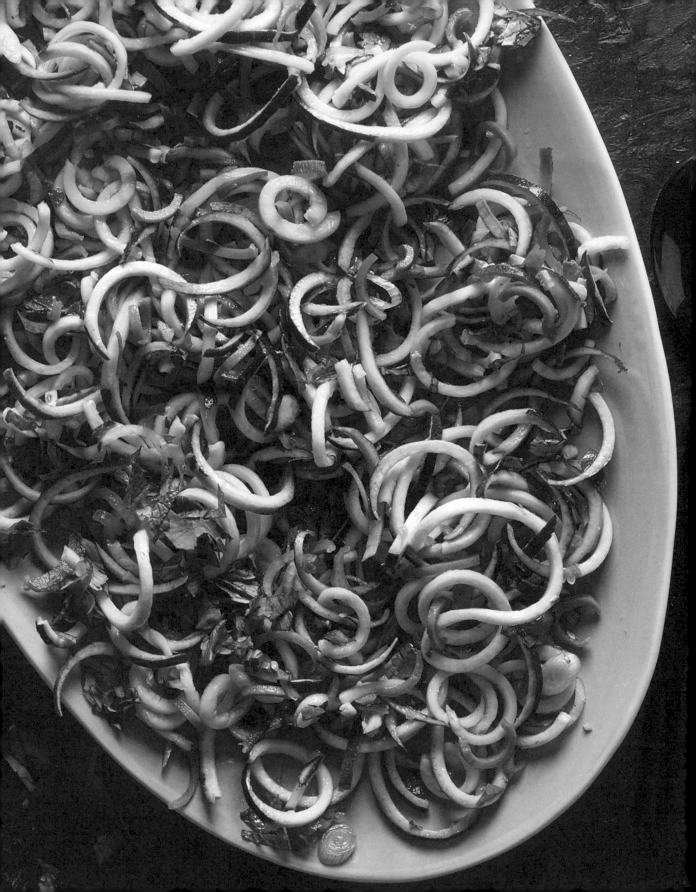

4 *Easy Vegetables and Sides*

Quick Pickled Red Onions

These pickled onions will be your new favorite condiment for the AIP and beyond. From salads to tacos, these onions add a pop of flavor and layer of complexity to every dish you add them to. Red onions boast an impressive nutrient profile: They are rich in antioxidants, contain cancer-fighting compounds, and have natural antibacterial properties. **MAKES 2 CUPS**

2 red onions, peeled
1 cup apple
  cider vinegar

2 tablespoons
  coconut sugar
1 tablespoon salt

**5-INGREDIENT
MAKE-AHEAD**

Prep time: 10 minutes
Pickling time: 24 hours

1. Slice the red onions ¼ inch thick and pack them into a pint-size Mason jar or other container with a tight-fitting lid.

2. In a small bowl, whisk together the vinegar, coconut sugar, and salt until the granules have dissolved.

3. Pour the vinegar mixture over the onions. Cover and refrigerate for up to 24 hours before eating (see Serving Tip).

Per Serving (2 tablespoons): Calories: 14; Total Fat: 0g; Saturated Fat: 0g; Sodium: 439mg; Carbohydrates: 3g; Fiber: 0g; Protein: 0g

Serving Tip: Though you can enjoy these onions in as little as 15 minutes, they are best when allowed to pickle for 24 hours or longer.

Ingredient Tip: You can use this recipe to pickle just about anything: Try pickled cucumbers, carrots, mango, or beets for a unique flavor addition to your diet. Get creative and add garlic or fresh herbs to the brine for different flavors to enjoy.

Make-Ahead Tip: In an airtight container, these onions can last for up to 1 month in the refrigerator. You can double, triple, or even quadruple this recipe depending on how much you use in a month.

Lemon Parsnip Hummus

Parsnips are root vegetables that look similar to white carrots. They have a very sweet and mild flavor with a slightly nutty taste, making them the perfect base for this AIP-friendly hummus. Parsnips are a great source of vitamins C and K, soluble and insoluble dietary fiber, antioxidants, and important micronutrients that may help support immune function. When puréed, these root vegetables make a perfectly smooth dip to enjoy with different vegetables or cold dishes. This hummus is excellent on sandwiches and wraps, and as a topping for raw salads. **MAKES 4 SERVINGS**

4 cups diced parsnips

4 garlic cloves

¼ cup sliced scallions, green and white parts

1 tablespoon chopped fresh parsley

1 tablespoon freshly squeezed lemon juice

1 tablespoon extra-virgin olive oil

1 teaspoon salt

5-INGREDIENT

30-MINUTE

Prep time: 5 minutes

Cook time: 20 minutes

1. Place the parsnips in a large saucepan and cover with cold water.

2. Bring the water to a rolling boil and allow to boil for 20 minutes, or until the parsnips are tender. Remove from the heat, drain the parsnips, and allow them to cool.

3. In a food processor, mince the garlic, scallions, and parsley for 30 seconds.

4. Add the parsnips, lemon juice, oil, and salt.

5. Purée for 1 to 2 minutes, stopping to scrape down the sides as needed, until the hummus is completely smooth.

Per Serving (½ cup): Calories: 137; Total Fat: 4g; Saturated Fat: 1g; Sodium: 597mg; Carbohydrates: 26g; Fiber: 7g; Protein: 2g

Ingredient Tip: Parsnips, garlic, lemon juice, olive oil, and salt form the base for this recipe, but you can easily swap in different fresh herbs for different taste combinations. Try using fresh basil, dill, or cilantro for new ways to enjoy this treat.

Serving Tip: Use this hummus as a dip for your favorite vegetables, as a spread for wraps in Grain-Free Tortillas (page 174), or as a condiment for sandwiches.

Beet and Mango Salsa

Replacing nightshades can be challenging when following the AIP, but luckily some small modifications and a little imagination can help create a tasty salsa that serves as a tasty dip or the perfect topping for fish or chicken, tacos or wraps, or hearty salads. Here, beets replace the tomatoes found in traditional salsa, providing many anti-inflammatory health benefits. **MAKES 4 SERVINGS**

1 cup diced
   cooked beets
1 cup diced avocado
1 cup diced mango
½ cup diced red onion
¼ cup chopped fresh
   cilantro

2 tablespoons white
   wine vinegar
1 tablespoon freshly
   squeezed lime juice
½ teaspoon salt

**30-MINUTE
ONE-BOWL**

Prep time: 10 minutes
Rest time: 10 minutes

1. In a large bowl, combine the beets, avocado, mango, onion, cilantro, vinegar, lime juice, and salt.

2. Stir well and allow to sit for 10 minutes before serving. Stir the salsa just before serving.

Per Serving (½ cup): Calories: 126; Total Fat: 7g; Saturated Fat: 1g; Sodium: 329mg; Carbohydrates: 17g; Fiber: 5g; Protein: 2g

Ingredient Tip: If the salsa is left to sit overnight, the color of the beets will seep into the other ingredients. Though the salsa will still taste good, the color will not be the same.

Serving Tip: Enjoy this salsa as a dip with Grain-Free Tortillas (page 174), or serve it with Mexican Cod Fish Tacos (page 80).

Creamy Pineapple Coleslaw

Coconut cream helps to create a creamy, tangy dressing for this classic staple salad. Both red and green cabbage have many important nutritional benefits, including prebiotic fibers that help feed the good gut bacteria in the digestive tract. Rich in vitamin C and vitamin K, cabbage also contains many inflammation-fighting nutrients and antioxidants like polyphenols and sulfur compounds. **MAKES 4 SERVINGS**

4 cups shredded
red and/or
green cabbage

1 cup diced pineapple

¼ cup coconut cream

¼ cup full-fat
coconut milk

1 tablespoon apple
cider vinegar

1 tablespoon
coconut sugar

¼ teaspoon ground
turmeric

¼ teaspoon salt

**30-MINUTE
ONE-BOWL**

Prep time: 10 minutes
Rest time: 20 minutes

1. In a large bowl, toss together the cabbage, pineapple, coconut cream, coconut milk, vinegar, coconut sugar, turmeric, and salt.

2. Allow the slaw to rest for 20 minutes before serving for the best flavor.

Per Serving (½ cup): Calories: 178; Total Fat: 14g; Saturated Fat: 11g; Sodium: 163mg; Carbohydrates: 14g; Fiber: 3g; Protein: 3g

Ingredient Tip: To save time and energy, you can purchase pre-shredded coleslaw mix from the grocery store. You can also purchase canned pineapple, as long as pineapple is the only ingredient listed on the label. Always purchase BPA-free canned products when possible.

Serving Tip: Enjoy this coleslaw as a delicious side dish with AIP-Friendly Fried Chicken (page 108) or Sheet Pan Lemon Haddock and Broccoli (page 81).

Dill and Radish Cucumber Salad

Radishes are a root vegetable with a definite crunchy texture and a sometimes spicy bite. Adding radishes to a salad is a perfect way to enjoy a burst of flavor and also get many nutritious health benefits. These little veggies contain dietary fiber and important nutrients like vitamin C, folic acid, potassium, zinc, phosphorus, and magnesium. They are also a great source of antioxidants and phytonutrients that can help support the immune system. **MAKES 4 SERVINGS**

1½ cups very thinly sliced radishes

1 cup very thinly sliced cucumber

1 tablespoon sliced scallion, green parts only

1 teaspoon chopped fresh dill

4 teaspoons extra-virgin olive oil

2 teaspoons freshly squeezed lemon juice

½ teaspoon salt

⅛ teaspoon coconut sugar

**30-MINUTE
ONE-BOWL**

Prep time: 10 minutes
Rest time: 15 minutes

Ingredient Tip: For a heartier salad, add 1 cup diced avocado. This will add more calories, heart-healthy fats, antioxidants, and nutrients.

1. In a medium bowl, combine the radishes, cucumber, scallion, dill, olive oil, lemon juice, salt, and coconut sugar. Stir well.

2. Enjoy right away or let the salad marinate for 15 minutes before serving to allow the flavors to fully develop.

Per Serving (½ cup): Calories: 53; Total Fat: 5g; Saturated Fat: 1g; Sodium: 309mg; Carbohydrates: 3g; Fiber: 1g; Protein: 1g

Balsamic Marinated Fennel Salad

Fennel is an underrated Mediterranean vegetable that offers a signature licorice flavor. Though the entire plant can be consumed, from the stalks to the seeds, for this recipe you only want to use the fennel bulb. The bulb offers an undeniable crunch in this fresh, flavor-packed salad. Fennel is highly nutritious, containing both soluble and insoluble forms of dietary fiber and important nutrients like potassium, calcium, and vitamins A and C. **MAKES 4 SERVINGS**

2 cups thinly sliced
    fennel (see
    Cooking Tip)
¼ cup balsamic vinegar

1 tablespoon
    extra-virgin olive oil
½ teaspoon sea salt

5-INGREDIENT
30-MINUTE
ONE-BOWL

Prep time: 10 minutes
Rest time: 20 minutes

1. In a medium bowl, combine the fennel, balsamic vinegar, olive oil, and sea salt. Toss well to coat.

2. Allow the salad to rest for 20 minutes before serving to fully develop the flavor.

Per Serving (½ cup): Calories: 47; Total Fat: 4g; Saturated Fat: 1g; Sodium: 257mg; Carbohydrates: 3g; Fiber: 1g; Protein: 1g

Cooking Tip: If you've never cooked with fennel before, the bulb may seem intimidating at first. To start, cut the top with the stems and stalks off and compost, discard, or save it for making Homemade Vegetable Bone Broth (page 162). Then, trim off the bottom, cut the bulb in half, and remove its tough middle core. Slice the bulb very thinly, like an onion.

Cold Asian Zoodle Salad

Herbs and spices are the secrets to delicious, flavorful meals on the AIP—just like in this recipe, where fresh herbs provide a bright pop of flavor and important nutrients that support overall health. Cilantro is a popular herb, praised for its ability to detox heavy metals from the blood; basil has naturally occurring anti-inflammatory properties; and mint has been shown to improve digestion and soothe stomach upset. **MAKES 4 SERVINGS**

2 tablespoons coconut liquid aminos

1 tablespoon extra-virgin olive oil

2 teaspoons freshly squeezed lime juice

1 teaspoon minced fresh gingerroot

½ teaspoon coconut sugar

4 cups spiralized zucchini

1 cup spiralized carrot

¼ cup spiralized radish

¼ cup sliced scallions, white and green parts

2 tablespoons chopped fresh cilantro

2 teaspoons chopped fresh basil (Thai basil if available)

2 teaspoons chopped fresh mint

30-MINUTE

Prep time: 20 minutes

Ingredient Tip: To make this recipe simpler, choose just one type of spiralized vegetable, such as zucchini noodles or carrot noodles. If you don't have a spiralizer, you can easily create veggie ribbons with a vegetable peeler. And don't forget to check your local grocery store to see if they have pre-spiralized vegetable noodles—this will cut down significantly on your prep time.

1. In a Mason jar or container with a tight-fitting lid, combine the aminos, olive oil, lime juice, ginger, and coconut sugar. Shake vigorously and set aside.

2. In a large bowl, toss together the spiralized vegetables, scallions, cilantro, basil, and mint.

3. Pour the dressing over the salad and mix well before serving.

Per Serving (½ cup): Calories: 75; Total Fat: 4g; Saturated Fat: 1g; Sodium: 43mg; Carbohydrates: 10g; Fiber: 2g; Protein: 2g

Shredded Brussels Sprout Salad

Although Brussels sprouts are usually consumed cooked, they can provide a unique texture to a cold, raw salad. This hearty shredded salad combines the tang of Brussels sprouts with the sweetness of carrots and cranberries to make a delicious accompaniment to any meal. These mini cruciferous vegetables are low in calories but high in vitamins and minerals, such as vitamins C and K. Vitamin K is an important nutrient for supporting both blood and bone health.

MAKES 4 SERVINGS

2 cups shredded
    Brussels sprouts
½ cup shredded carrots
¼ cup unsweetened
    dried cranberries

¼ cup Apple Cider
    Vinaigrette
    (page 170)

5-INGREDIENT
30-MINUTE
ONE-BOWL

Prep time: 10 minutes
Rest time: 10 minutes

1. In a large bowl, toss together the Brussels sprouts, carrots, cranberries, and vinaigrette.

2. Allow the salad to sit for 10 minutes; toss again just before serving.

Per Serving (½ cup): Calories: 145; Total Fat: 12g; Saturated Fat: 2g; Sodium: 112mg; Carbohydrates: 9g; Fiber: 2g; Protein: 2g

Ingredient Tip: If you can, purchase pre-shredded Brussels sprouts from the grocery store. This will cut down your prep time considerably. You can also purchase matchstick carrots, making this truly a five-minute salad to put together.

Serving Tip: Use this salad as a base for a more substantial entrée-style meal by topping it with Slow Cooker Shredded Chicken (page 107).

Cinnamon Baked Sweet Potato Chips

Everyone craves a crunchy snack once in a while. That's where these baked sweet potato chips come in. You can make them either sweet or savory, and they are sure to satisfy that afternoon snack craving. Sweet potatoes are commonly mistaken for a nightshade, but they are not, making them an excellent choice for the AIP. These nutrient-dense root tubers are most known for their abundance of antioxidants—especially beta-carotene, a compound that is turned into vitamin A by the body and is responsible for the vegetable's bright orange color.

MAKES 4 SERVINGS

2 large sweet potatoes
1 teaspoon extra-virgin
 olive oil
½ teaspoon ground
 cinnamon
½ teaspoon salt

5-INGREDIENT

Prep time: 10 minutes
Cook time: 35 minutes

1. Preheat the oven to 400°F. Line one or two baking sheets with aluminum foil, top with a wire baking rack, and set aside.
2. Using a mandoline or sharp knife, carefully cut the sweet potato into ⅛-inch-thick slices.
3. Toss the sweet potato slices with the olive oil and cinnamon.
4. Arrange the sweet potato slices evenly on the baking rack(s) set on the baking sheet(s), spreading out the pieces as much as possible. Sprinkle with the salt.
5. Bake the chips for 25 to 30 minutes, or until crispy.
6. Allow to cool for 5 minutes before serving.

Ingredient Tip: This recipe can be made with all different types of root vegetables. Try carrot chips, parsnip chips, or even beet chips. For a savory chip, swap out the ground cinnamon for ground ginger or your favorite AIP-approved spice.

Per Serving (1 cup): Calories: 81; Total Fat: 1g; Saturated Fat: 0g; Sodium: 335mg; Carbohydrates: 17g; Fiber: 3g; Protein: 1g

Baked Rutabaga French Fries

Rutabagas are another root vegetable that quickly becomes an AIP staple. The white veggie has a starchy consistency that makes it a perfect substitute for white potatoes. Rich in vitamin C and other oxidant-fighting and immune-supporting nutrients, rutabagas are a nutritious addition to any diet. They also contains manganese, potassium, thiamin, vitamin B$_6$, calcium, magnesium, and phosphorus.

MAKES 4 SERVINGS

1½ pounds rutabagas
1 tablespoon
    extra-virgin olive oil
1 teaspoon AIP Spice
    Blend (page 160)
Salt

5-INGREDIENT

Prep time: 10 minutes
Cook time: 45 minutes

1. Preheat the oven to 450°F. Line a baking sheet with aluminum foil.

2. Using a chef's knife, carefully peel off the outside skin of the rutabagas.

3. Slice the rutabagas into ½-by-2-inch sticks, resembling French fries.

4. In a large bowl, toss the rutabagas with the olive oil.

5. Spread the rutabagas on the prepared baking sheet, sprinkle with the spice blend and salt to taste, and bake for 45 minutes, or until golden brown and crispy, flipping once halfway through.

Cooking Tip: If you have an oven with a convection bake setting, use it set at the same temperature. This will yield crispier fries. Don't forget to serve these with AIP-Friendly Ketchup (page 161).

Per Serving (1 cup): Calories: 91; Total Fat: 4g; Saturated Fat: 1g; Sodium: 160mg; Carbohydrates: 14g; Fiber: 4g; Protein: 2g

Savory Pumpkin Gnocchi

One thing many clients miss while on the AIP is a hearty, filling pasta meal, and these savory gnocchi bites are one of the closest ways to satisfy that craving. Traditionally reserved for pie, pumpkin is a sweet fruit that has many nutritional similarities to vegetables like winter squash. The bright orange color signifies the antioxidants beta-carotene, alpha-carotene, and beta-cryptoxanthin, all of which fight free radicals in the body. **MAKES 4 SERVINGS**

1 (15-ounce) can
   pumpkin purée
1½ cups cassava flour
1 tablespoon
   nutritional yeast
½ teaspoon salt

½ teaspoon
   garlic powder
3 tablespoons
   extra-virgin olive oil
   (optional)
1 tablespoon chopped
   fresh sage (optional)

**5-INGREDIENT
MAKE-AHEAD**

Prep time: 30 minutes
Cook time: 30 minutes

Make-Ahead Tip: Once all of the gnocchi are made, you can freeze them in individual portion–size bags. When ready to use, remove the gnocchi from the freezer and proceed from step 6.

Ingredient Tip: Check the canned pumpkin's ingredients label to ensure that there are no additives.

1. Place a large stockpot of water on the stove to boil.

2. In a large bowl, combine the pumpkin, flour, nutritional yeast, salt, and garlic powder. Mix well with a spatula until a dough is formed.

3. Using your hands, shape handfuls of dough into long cylinders, about the thickness of a roll of quarters.

4. Use a knife to cut the cylinders of dough into ½-inch pieces, resembling gnocchi. Place the cut dough pieces on a sheet of parchment paper.

5. After all of the pieces are cut, either leave them as they are for a rustic look, or roll each piece down the back of a fork to get classic gnocchi-shaped ridges.

6. Drop the shaped gnocchi into the boiling water and cook for 3 to 5 minutes, or until they float to the top.

7. Drain the gnocchi in a colander, or use a slotted spoon to scoop the pieces out of the water, and return them to the parchment paper.

8. Serve the gnocchi as is with your favorite sauce, or proceed to the next step and sauté them.

9. Optional step: Warm the olive oil in a large skillet over medium-high heat. Once the oil is hot, add the gnocchi. Let one side brown for 1 to 2 minutes, flip, and then let the other side brown for 1 to 2 minutes. Sprinkle with the sage and cook for 1 more minute before serving.

Per Serving (½ cup): Calories: 213; Total Fat: 1g; Saturated Fat: 0g; Sodium: 489mg; Carbohydrates: 48g; Fiber: 10g; Protein: 4g

From-Scratch Cauliflower Rice

Cauliflower rice is a popular staple among those who follow a grain-free diet, and for good reason. Its mild flavor and unique texture make it perfect for "ricing." High in dietary fiber and antioxidants, cauliflower contains many powerful plant compounds that reduce the risk of disease. Cauliflower also contains many important nutrients like folate, potassium, magnesium, and phosphorus, as well as vitamins C, K, and B$_6$. **MAKES 4 SERVINGS**

½ cup chopped
   yellow onion
1 teaspoon
   minced garlic
8 cups cauliflower
   florets

1 tablespoon
   extra-virgin olive oil
½ teaspoon salt
   (optional)

**5-INGREDIENT
30-MINUTE**

Prep time: 10 minutes
Cook time: 10 minutes

1. In a food processor, pulse the yellow onion and garlic for 30 to 60 seconds, or until finely minced.

2. Add the cauliflower florets and pulse in 15-second intervals to break down the pieces. Stop often to scrape down the sides, as you do not want to create a cauliflower purée. Continue pulsing until all the cauliflower is broken down into rice-size pieces.

3. Heat the olive oil in a skillet over medium heat.

4. Add the ingredients from the food processor and sauté for approximately 5 minutes, stirring occasionally, until the cauliflower is just tender.

5. Cover and cook for an additional 3 minutes before serving. Season with salt if you like.

Per Serving (½ cup): Calories: 87; Total Fat: 4g; Saturated Fat: 1g; Sodium: 351mg; Carbohydrates: 12g; Fiber: 5g; Protein: 4g

Ingredient Tip: Though it's helpful to know how to make cauliflower rice from scratch, you can usually purchase riced cauliflower from the grocery store. Some stores carry fresh cauliflower rice, and some stores carry frozen—just check the ingredients list to ensure that no other ingredients have been added.

Baked Herbed Zucchini Boats

Zucchini is a hearty vegetable that makes the perfect base for many different entrée-style dishes. Baked zucchini boats can be filled with a combination of different meats and vegetables for a substantial meal. These summer squash are low in calories but contain important nutrients like vitamins C and K, folate, riboflavin, potassium, and manganese. Packed with antioxidants and phytonutrients, zucchini can help improve digestion and regulate blood sugar levels, and they may even support thyroid function. **MAKES 4 SERVINGS**

2 large zucchini
1 tablespoon
    extra-virgin olive oil
1 teaspoon AIP Spice
    Blend (page 160)

5-INGREDIENT
30-MINUTE
ONE-PAN

Prep time: 10 minutes
Cook time: 20 minutes

1. Preheat the oven to 400°F. Line a baking sheet with aluminum foil and set aside.

2. Cut the zucchini in half lengthwise and scoop out the seeds, creating a well that runs down the center of the zucchini half. Place on the prepared baking sheet.

3. Brush the inside of each half with the olive oil and evenly sprinkle with the spice blend.

4. Bake flat-side up for 20 to 25 minutes, or until fork-tender.

Per Serving (1 zucchini boat): Calories: 56; Total Fat: 4g; Saturated Fat: 1g; Sodium: 76mg; Carbohydrates: 5g; Fiber: 2g; Protein: 2g

Ingredient Tip: You can swap out zucchini for yellow squash. You can also substitute different fresh herbs and spices, as long as they are AIP-friendly, to create new flavor combinations.

Serving Tip: For a satisfying comfort food meal, try filling one of these zucchini boats with Slow Cooker Shredded Chicken (page 107) and some Cauliflower Alfredo Sauce (page 166).

Sautéed Lemon Garlic Kale

Kale, one of today's most popular and versatile dark leafy greens, is a member of the cruciferous vegetable family. This superfood contains many nutrients that help support the body during times of healing and repair. Kale is packed with dietary fiber, vitamins A, C, and K, and alpha-linolenic acid, an omega-3 fatty acid. **MAKES 4 SERVINGS**

2 tablespoons
   extra-virgin olive oil
8 cups chopped
   kale leaves
½ teaspoon salt

2 teaspoons
   minced garlic
1½ tablespoons freshly
   squeezed lemon juice

5-INGREDIENT
30-MINUTE
ONE-POT

Prep time: 10 minutes
Cook time: 10 minutes

1. Heat a large skillet over medium-high heat.

2. When the skillet is hot, carefully add the olive oil and swirl to coat the entire bottom.

3. Add the kale and sprinkle with the salt. Sauté for 5 to 7 minutes, stirring constantly, until the kale is wilted.

4. Stir in the garlic and cook for an additional 2 minutes.

5. Add the lemon juice, stir well, and serve.

Ingredient Tip: The chopped kale can be swapped out for any dark leafy green like spinach or collard greens. Additionally, if you find mature kale to be too tough and fibrous for your preference, opt for baby kale instead, which is softer and much milder.

Per Serving (½ cup): Calories: 131; Total Fat: 7g; Saturated Fat: 1g; Sodium: 351mg; Carbohydrates: 15g; Fiber: 2g; Protein: 4g

Sautéed Zoodles in Alfredo Sauce

Zoodles are simply zucchini that have been spiralized into noodle form. Both zucchini and yellow squash are packed with dietary fiber and beneficial nutrients like vitamins A and C and minerals like potassium and folate. Even people on unrestricted diets agree that zoodles make an excellent substitution for pasta in traditional dishes like this. **MAKES 4 SERVINGS**

4 zucchini or yellow
    squash, spiralized
    (see Ingredient Tip)
½ teaspoon salt
1 tablespoon
    extra-virgin olive oil

1 teaspoon
    minced garlic
1 cup Cauliflower
    Alfredo Sauce
    (page 166)

**5-INGREDIENT
30-MINUTE**

Prep time: 10 minutes
Cook time: 15 minutes

1. Place the spiralized zucchini in a colander with the salt and allow it to drain for 10 minutes.

2. In a large nonstick skillet, heat the olive oil over medium heat. Add the garlic and sauté for 1 minute, or until fragrant.

3. Add the zoodles to the pan and cook, stirring frequently, for 2 minutes, or until heated through.

4. Add the alfredo sauce to the pan and heat for 1 minute, tossing with the zoodles to coat well.

Ingredient Tip: If you don't have a spiralizer, you can simply use a vegetable peeler to create zucchini ribbons. You can also create zoodles or ribbons from yellow summer squash or carrots.

Per Serving (½ cup): Calories: 90; Total Fat: 4g; Saturated Fat: 1g; Sodium: 440mg; Carbohydrates: 10g; Fiber: 3g; Protein: 4g

Balsamic Roasted Mushrooms

Mushrooms are considered a superfood because of their high nutrient content and extraordinary health benefits. Many types of mushrooms are available at the market today, but most carry the same nutritious benefits. Some of the most important nutrients found in mushrooms are B vitamins, selenium, potassium, and vitamin D. The prebiotic content in mushrooms can help boost your immune system and improve digestion. **MAKES 4 SERVINGS**

2 tablespoons
   extra-virgin olive oil
¼ cup balsamic vinegar
1 tablespoon
   minced garlic

½ teaspoon salt
1½ pounds whole
   cremini mushrooms,
   stems trimmed
1 red onion, thinly sliced

**5-INGREDIENT
30-MINUTE**

Prep time: 10 minutes
Cook time: 20 minutes

1. Preheat the oven to 400°F.

2. In a Mason jar, combine the olive oil, vinegar, garlic, and salt. Tightly fasten the top and shake vigorously to combine. Set aside.

3. In a large bowl, combine the mushrooms and red onion.

4. Pour the balsamic mixture over the mushroom mixture, and stir until well coated.

5. Transfer the mushrooms and onion to a 9-by-13-inch baking dish. Bake for 20 minutes, stirring once halfway through.

Cooking Tip: When preparing the baking dish, try to arrange your mushrooms stem-side down to help them release some of their moisture during the cooking process.

Per Serving (½ cup): Calories: 120; Total Fat: 7g; Saturated Fat: 1g; Sodium: 293mg; Carbohydrates: 10g; Fiber: 1g; Protein: 5g

Herbed Whole Roasted Cauliflower

Cauliflower, a good source of antioxidants, also contains vitamins C, K, and B$_6$, as well as potassium and magnesium. When cooked whole, it becomes soft and buttery on the inside yet remains crispy and perfectly golden brown on the outside. **MAKES 4 SERVINGS**

Olive oil cooking spray

2 small heads cauliflower

2 tablespoons extra-virgin olive oil

1 tablespoon minced garlic

1 tablespoon AIP Spice Blend (page 160)

1 teaspoon salt

5-INGREDIENT
ONE-PAN

Prep time: 10 minutes
Cook time: 1 hour

1. Preheat the oven to 350°F. Lightly grease a baking dish or Dutch oven with cooking spray.

2. Remove the outer leaves of the cauliflower and cut a slice off the bottom so it will sit upright in the pan. Place the cauliflower, core-side down, inside the baking dish.

3. Using your hands or a brush, coat the head of cauliflower with the olive oil and minced garlic.

4. Sprinkle evenly with the spice blend and salt.

5. Cover the baking dish with a lid or aluminum foil and bake for 45 minutes, or until it is easily pierced with a sharp knife.

6. Uncover and bake for another 15 minutes, or until the outside is nicely browned.

7. Carefully remove the cauliflower from the oven. To serve, slice the whole head lengthwise to create slabs or cauliflower "steaks," or cut it into wedges the size of cake slices.

Ingredient Tip: This recipe can be done with a head of broccoli, too. Whether you use cauliflower or broccoli, you'll have a blank canvas for any flavor you choose. Try swapping the AIP Spice Blend for another approved spice, or use some chopped fresh herbs like parsley or basil.

Serving Tip: Serve this as an accompaniment to meat-based entrées, or enjoy a cauliflower "steak" as a plant-based main dish along with other sides.

Per Serving (½ roasted cauliflower): Calories: 96; Total Fat: 7g; Saturated Fat: 1g; Sodium: 621mg; Carbohydrates: 8g; Fiber: 3g; Protein: 3g

Roasted Spaghetti Squash Bowls

Spaghetti squash is a pretty magical vegetable that produces spaghetti-like strands when cooked, making it another excellent pasta replacement for those following a grain-free diet. Unlike other winter squash varieties, spaghetti squash is low in carbohydrates. It's also rich in B vitamins such as riboflavin, niacin, and thiamin, and it contains omega-3s, the fatty acids associated with reduced inflammation. **MAKES 4 SERVINGS**

2 small spaghetti squash
1 teaspoon extra-virgin
   olive oil
1 teaspoon AIP Spice
   Blend (page 160)
¼ teaspoon salt

**5-INGREDIENT
ONE-PAN**

Prep time: 10 minutes
Cook time: 45 minutes

1. Preheat the oven to 400°F (convention bake if available). Line a baking sheet with aluminum foil.

2. Cut the spaghetti squash in half lengthwise and scoop out the seeds. Lay each spaghetti squash half flat-side up on the prepared baking sheet.

3. Drizzle each half with olive oil and evenly season with the spice blend and salt. Bake for 45 minutes, or until the squash is easily pierced with a fork.

4. Allow to cool for 5 minutes before using a fork to gently release the strands from the rind.

Serving Tip: Serve Creamy Chicken Florentine (page 110) or Slow Cooker Shredded Chicken (page 107) directly inside the spaghetti squash bowl for a hearty, no-mess meal.

Per Serving (½ cup): Calories: 73; Total Fat: 2g; Saturated Fat: 0g; Sodium: 345mg; Carbohydrates: 14g; Fiber: 0g; Protein: 1g

Hasselback Baked Sweet Potatoes

A delicious comfort food, baked sweet potatoes offer more nutrients and a sweeter taste than traditional white potatoes. Sweet potatoes are high in dietary fiber, and they pair well with health-promoting, warming spices like cinnamon. Cinnamon is loaded with antioxidants and has many medicinal and anti-inflammatory properties that have been used for centuries. The hasselback style of preparing this dish allows for a new, crispier texture and fun presentation. See the Ingredient Tip for a savory preparation option. **MAKES 4 SERVINGS**

4 sweet potatoes
1 tablespoon
    coconut oil
1 tablespoon
    coconut sugar

½ teaspoon ground
    cinnamon
½ teaspoon salt

5-INGREDIENT

Prep time: 10 minutes
Cook time: 45 minutes

1. Preheat the oven to 400°F. Line a baking sheet with aluminum foil.

2. To make hasselback-style potatoes, slice a very small layer off the bottom of each potato to keep it from rolling around.

3. Then, create ⅛-inch-thick vertical cuts along the sweet potato, being careful not to cut through the bottom (leave a ¼-inch-thick base).

4. In a small bowl, mix together the coconut oil, coconut sugar, cinnamon, and salt.

continued

Ingredient Tip: Omit the coconut sugar and ground cinnamon if you don't want a sweet flavor profile for this dish. Instead, try topping it with the AIP Spice Blend (page 160) for a savory version.

Cooking Tip: To make cutting the hasselback potato easier, get two wooden spoons and place one handle on each side of the sweet potato. This will help you keep the base of the potato intact as you cut the vertical slices.

5. Brush half of the oil mixture over the sweet potatoes and place them on the prepared baking sheet.

6. Bake for 45 minutes, or until tender.

7. Just before serving, brush the potatoes with the remaining oil mixture.

Per Serving (1 potato): Calories: 153; Total Fat: 4g; Saturated Fat: 3g; Sodium: 362mg; Carbohydrates: 29g; Fiber: 4g; Protein: 2g

Garlic Mashed Rutabagas

A rutabaga, often confused for a turnip, is a mellow-tasting root vegetable that substitutes well for the traditional white potato. In the case of classic mashed potatoes, rutabagas are an excellent swap because they are not a nightshade vegetable but have a look and feel similar to mashed potatoes when cooked and mashed—plus, they contain powerful antioxidants. **MAKES 4 SERVINGS**

4 cups peeled and
    diced rutabagas
4 garlic cloves
1 teaspoon salt

2 cups filtered water
2 teaspoons extra-virgin
    olive oil

**5-INGREDIENT
30-MINUTE**

Prep time: 10 minutes
Cook time: 20 minutes

1. In a medium saucepan, combine the rutabagas, garlic, salt, and water.

2. Cover the pan, bring the water to a boil, and allow to boil for 5 minutes.

3. Reduce the heat to low and simmer for 30 minutes, or until the rutabagas are soft and fork-tender.

4. Drain the rutabagas and transfer to a food processor.

5. Add the olive oil, cover tightly, and purée until the mixture reaches your desired consistency.

Cooking Tip: If you have an immersion blender, you can use it to purée the rutabaga in the same pan it cooks in. Or, if you like a chunkier texture, you can mash the rutabagas by hand with a potato masher.

Per Serving (½ cup): Calories: 75; Total Fat: 3g; Saturated Fat: 0g; Sodium: 610mg; Carbohydrates: 12g; Fiber: 4g; Protein: 2g

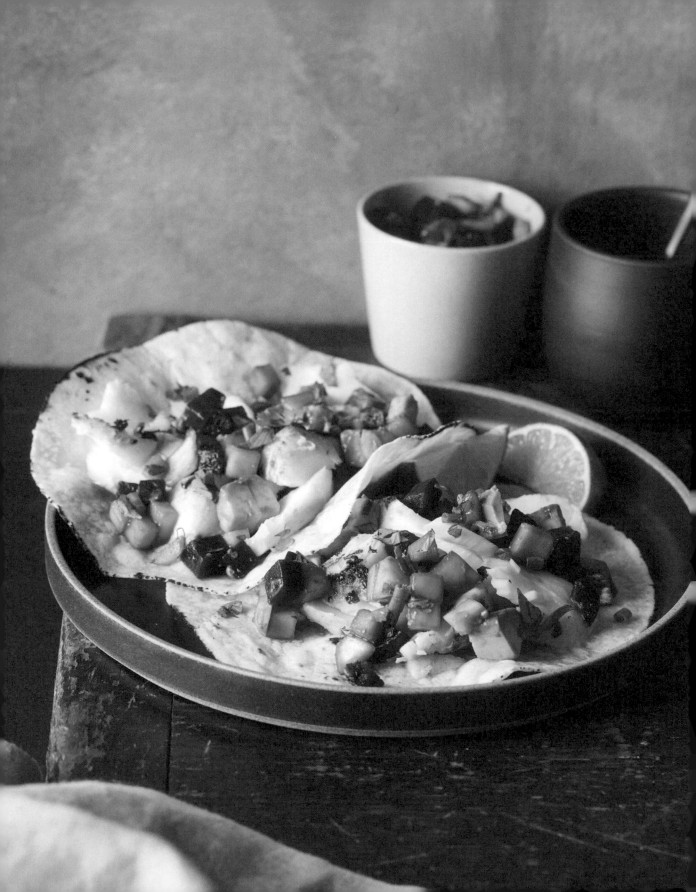

5 *Seafood Mains*

Chilled Mango Salmon Salad Wraps

Canned or individually packed salmon is a wonderfully beneficial convenience food for those following the AIP. Just ensure that the ingredients contain nothing but wild-caught salmon, olive oil, and salt, and you'll have a high-quality seafood product that requires no preparation or cook time. Using canned fish helps this dish come together in just a few minutes, while still providing the important nutrients and heart-healthy fats supplied by wild-caught salmon.

MAKES 4 SERVINGS

2 (6-ounce) cans
   wild-caught salmon in
   olive oil, drained
1 avocado, pitted
   and diced
½ cup finely
   diced mango

¼ cup diced red onion
2 tablespoons
   coconut cream
½ teaspoon salt
4 Grain-Free Tortillas
   (page 174)
1 cup spring mix

**30-MINUTE
ONE-BOWL**

Prep time: 10 minutes
Rest time: 10 minutes

Ingredient Tip: No fresh tortillas on hand? No problem—enjoy this salad over a bed of spring mix instead.

1. In a medium bowl, gently mash the drained salmon with a fork.

2. Add the avocado, mango, red onion, coconut cream, and salt. Mash with a fork until all ingredients are well combined and the avocado is no longer chunky.

3. Refrigerate for 10 minutes before serving to chill the salad and develop the flavors.

4. Scoop one-quarter of the salmon salad into each tortilla, top with the spring mix, roll up, and serve.

Per Serving (1 wrap): Calories: 316; Total Fat: 15g; Saturated Fat: 14g; Sodium: 632mg; Carbohydrates: 22g; Fiber: 6g; Protein: 21g

Cranberry Salmon Spinach Salad

This quick and easy salad is a nutrient powerhouse. Spinach is packed with dietary fiber, vitamins C and K, folic acid, iron, and calcium, as well as important B vitamins. Salmon is also abundant in nutrients and omega-3 fatty acids. The delicate flavor of the spinach pairs well with the tart cranberries and savory salmon in this colorful, entrée-style salad. **MAKES 4 SERVINGS**

1 pound wild-caught
    salmon, cut into
    4 (4-ounce) fillets
1 teaspoon sea salt
6 cups baby spinach
1 cup diced orange
    segments
    (1-inch pieces)

½ cup unsweetened
    dried cranberries
½ cup Sweet Beet
    Vinaigrette
    (page 169)

5-INGREDIENT
30-MINUTE

Prep time: 10 minutes
Cook time: 15 minutes

Ingredient Tip: Don't have time to cook? Swap in canned salmon for an even quicker and easier lunch. Omit the salmon fillets and opt for 2 (6-ounce) cans of wild-caught salmon in olive oil, drained.

1. Preheat the oven to 450°F. Line a baking sheet with parchment paper and set aside.

2. Season both sides of the salmon fillets with the sea salt.

3. Place the fillets skin-side down on the prepared baking sheet. Bake for 12 to 15 minutes, or until the salmon has reached an internal temperature of 145°F.

4. Meanwhile, divide the spinach evenly among 4 bowls. Top with the orange pieces and cranberries.

5. When the salmon is cooked through (it should flake easily with a fork), remove it from the oven and place one fillet on top of each salad.

6. Drizzle with the vinaigrette and enjoy.

Per Serving (1 salad): Calories: 496; Total Fat: 37g; Saturated Fat: 6g; Sodium: 720mg; Carbohydrates: 16g; Fiber: 3g; Protein: 29g

Orange Ginger Roasted Salmon

Salmon is a popular fatty fish that has been shown to help reduce inflammation in the body thanks to its EPA and DHA omega-3 fatty acids. Salmon is also a good source of high-quality protein and B vitamins, such as thiamin, riboflavin, and niacin. Although some people find the taste of salmon strong, many love it, and the orange and ginger in this recipe help balance the flavors and make this a truly delicious dish the whole family will enjoy. **MAKES 4 SERVINGS**

¼ cup raw honey

¼ cup freshly squeezed orange juice

2 tablespoons freshly squeezed lemon juice

2 garlic cloves, roughly chopped

1½-inch piece fresh gingerroot, peeled and thinly sliced

1 pound wild-caught salmon, cut into 4 (4-ounce) fillets

Salt

30-MINUTE

Prep time: 20 minutes
Cook time: 10 minutes

Cooking Tip: This recipe can also be made on the grill if you're cooking outdoors.

1. Preheat the oven to 325°F. Line a baking sheet with aluminum foil and set aside.

2. In a small saucepan over medium heat, combine the honey, orange juice, lemon juice, garlic, and ginger. Cook, stirring occasionally, until the liquid just comes to a boil.

3. Remove the marinade from the stovetop and strain the solids, retaining the liquid. Set the liquid aside to cool.

4. Place the salmon fillets in a shallow container and cover with three-quarters of the marinade. Let sit 10 minutes. Reserve the remaining marinade for basting.

5. Place the salmon fillets skin-side down on the prepared baking sheet. Season liberally with salt.

6. Bake the salmon for 7 minutes.

7. Remove the salmon from the oven and brush with the remaining marinade. Increase the oven temperature to broil.

8. Place the salmon under the broiler for 2 to 3 minutes, or until the glaze begins to caramelize. Watch closely to prevent overcooking.

9. Remove from the oven and serve immediately.

Per Serving (1 fillet): Calories: 335; Total Fat: 18g; Saturated Fat: 4g; Sodium: 101mg; Carbohydrates: 22g; Fiber: 1g; Protein: 22g

Greek Salmon en Papillote

En papillote is a French term for cooking in parchment. This style of cooking is simple and easily customizable for a variety of seafood dishes. For this recipe, you'll use parchment paper to create your pouch for cooking. The fish is steamed and poached in the parchment, resulting in a moist and flaky fillet with tender, perfectly cooked vegetables. **MAKES 4 SERVINGS**

1 pound wild-caught Alaskan sockeye salmon, cut into 4 (4-ounce) fillets

2 teaspoons minced fresh oregano

1 teaspoon salt

2 medium zucchini, cut into thin strips

2 medium yellow squash, cut into thin strips

1 cup sliced white onion

¼ cup freshly squeezed lemon juice

2 tablespoons minced garlic

2 tablespoons extra-virgin olive oil

30-MINUTE
ONE-PAN

Prep time: 10 minutes
Cook time: 15 minutes

Substitution Tip: This recipe easily works with milder seafood options like tilapia, cod, haddock, or even shrimp.

1. Preheat the oven to 400°F.

2. To prepare each packet (you will need two), tear off a large sheet of parchment paper and fold it in half. Fold over two of the edges, creating a tight seam. Fold multiple times if needed, but leave one side open.

3. Season the salmon fillets with the oregano and salt. Place 2 fillets in each parchment packet.

4. Divide the zucchini, yellow squash, white onion, lemon juice, garlic, and olive oil evenly between the two packets.

5. Seal the remaining open side of each parchment packet tightly by folding it over on itself several times.

6. Place the packets on a baking sheet and bake for 15 minutes, or until the salmon is flaky and has reached an internal temperature of 145°F.

7. Evenly divide the contents of each packet into 4 servings.

Per Serving (1 fillet, 1 cup vegetables): Calories: 327; Total Fat: 17g; Saturated Fat: 3g; Sodium: 536mg; Carbohydrates: 12g; Fiber: 3g; Protein: 32g

Mahi-Mahi with Mango Agrodolce

Mahi-mahi is a tropical fish that is exceptionally rich in the omega-3 fatty acids that help reduce inflammation in the body. "Mahi," as it's also called, is high in protein and vitamins B_3 and B_6, along with many powerful antioxidants. Finished with Mango Agrodolce (page 168), an Italian sweet-and-sour sauce, this sweet main dish has tropical flair. **MAKES 4 SERVINGS**

Olive oil cooking spray
1 pound mahi-mahi, cut into 4 (4-ounce) fillets
¼ teaspoon salt
1 tablespoon coconut liquid aminos

1 teaspoon extra-virgin olive oil
½ teaspoon coconut sugar
½ cup Mango Agrodolce (page 168)

5-INGREDIENT
30-MINUTE

Prep time: 10 minutes
Cook time: 20 minutes

Substitution Tip: If you don't have any Mango Agrodolce made, this dish is also excellent topped with Beet and Mango Salsa (page 50).

1. Preheat the oven to 400°F. Spray a baking dish with cooking spray and set it aside.

2. Season both sides of the mahi-mahi with the salt. Place it in the prepared baking dish.

3. In a small bowl, whisk together the aminos, olive oil, and coconut sugar. Pour the mixture over the fish and let marinate for 10 minutes.

4. Bake the fish for 13 to 15 minutes, or until it flakes easily with a fork and reaches an internal temperature of 145°F.

5. Top with the agrodolce just before serving.

Per Serving (1 fillet): Calories: 201; Total Fat: 3g; Saturated Fat: 1g; Sodium: 571mg; Carbohydrates: 9g; Fiber: 1g; Protein: 31g

Pan-Roasted Halibut

Pan roasting is a two-step method that involves cooking on high heat on the stove, then cooking at a lower temperature in the oven to produce a crispy outside and a tender inside. You can pan roast just about anything; in this case, pan roasting brings out the halibut's delicate flavor. **MAKES 4 SERVINGS**

1 pound wild-caught halibut, cut into 4 (4-ounce) fillets
¼ teaspoon salt
2 tablespoons extra-virgin olive oil
1 teaspoon thyme
1 teaspoon dill
8 fresh chives
2 tablespoons coconut butter

5-INGREDIENT
30-MINUTE
ONE-POT

Prep time: 5 minutes
Cook time: 20 minutes

1. Preheat the oven to 350°F.
2. Rinse the halibut and pat it dry with a clean towel.
3. Season both sides of the dry fillets with the salt.
4. Heat the olive oil in an oven-safe skillet over medium-high heat.
5. When the oil is hot, add the halibut fillets to the skillet and cook on one side for 3 to 4 minutes.
6. Gently flip the fillets and top them with the fresh herbs and coconut butter.
7. When the butter melts, use a spoon to gently baste the halibut for 1 minute.
8. Transfer the entire pan to the preheated oven. Cook 4 minutes for medium-rare, 9 minutes for well done.
9. Remove the pan from the oven and baste the fillets with the butter and herb mixture.
10. Let the fish rest for 2 to 3 minutes before serving topped with the herbs and butter.

Per Serving (1 fillet): Calories: 298; Total Fat: 19g; Saturated Fat: 10g; Sodium: 228mg; Carbohydrates: 4g; Fiber: 3g; Protein: 30g

Mexican Cod Fish Tacos

Enjoy this mild, flaky fish in a classic favorite presentation: fish tacos. A naturally low-fat fish, cod is a good source of protein and is packed with important nutrients like phosphorus and vitamin B_{12}. It pairs well with the bold flavors of fresh lime and cilantro in this Mexican-inspired dish. **MAKES 4 SERVINGS**

1 pound cod fish, cut into 4 (4-ounce) fillets
½ teaspoon salt, divided
½ teaspoon garlic powder
1 teaspoon chopped fresh cilantro
1 teaspoon chopped fresh chives

2 teaspoons extra-virgin olive oil
8 Grain-Free Tortillas (page 174)
1 cup Creamy Pineapple Coleslaw (page 51)

**30-MINUTE
ONE-PAN**

Prep time: 5 minutes
Cook time: 10 minutes

Ingredient Tip: This recipe is flexible, so feel free to swap out the cod for other flaky white fish such as haddock or flounder.

1. Preheat the oven broiler to high. Line a baking sheet with aluminum foil.

2. Lay the cod fillets on the prepared baking sheet and top each fillet with one-quarter each of the salt, garlic powder, cilantro, and chives.

3. Drizzle each fillet evenly with the olive oil.

4. Place the fish under the broiler and cook for 5 to 7 minutes, or until it reaches an internal temperature of 135°F and flakes easily with a fork.

5. Break the fish into flakes and enjoy it inside the tortillas topped with the coleslaw (2 tablespoons slaw per taco).

Per Serving (2 fish tacos): Calories: 314; Total Fat: 12g; Saturated Fat: 6g; Sodium: 761mg; Carbohydrates: 31g; Fiber: 6g; Protein: 22g

Sheet Pan Lemon Haddock and Broccoli

Haddock is a mild, flaky white fish loaded with B vitamins and minerals like selenium, magnesium, and niacin as well as heart-healthy omega 3-fatty acids.

MAKES 4 SERVINGS

4 cups broccoli florets
1 tablespoon
    extra-virgin olive oil
1 teaspoon AIP
    Spice Blend
    (page 160), divided

1 teaspoon kosher
    salt, divided
1 pound wild-caught
    haddock, cut into
    4 (4-ounce) fillets
1 lemon, thinly sliced

5-INGREDIENT
30-MINUTE
ONE-PAN

Prep time: 5 minutes
Cook time: 25 minutes

Ingredient Tip: This recipe can easily be made with other white fish such as cod, flounder, or trout.

1. Preheat the oven to 350°F. Line a baking sheet with aluminum foil or parchment paper.

2. Spread the broccoli florets on the prepared baking sheet and drizzle with the olive oil. Sprinkle with ½ teaspoon of spice blend and ½ teaspoon of salt.

3. Using a spatula, gently toss the broccoli to coat. Bake for 15 minutes, or until the broccoli is just tender.

4. Meanwhile, season the haddock fillets with the remaining ½ teaspoon each of spice blend and salt.

5. Remove the baking sheet from the oven and carefully push the broccoli to the outside perimeter of the pan. Place the haddock fillets in the center.

6. Top the fish with the lemon slices and return the baking sheet to the oven until the haddock is light and flaky and has reached an internal temperature of 145°F, about 10 minutes. Serve immediately.

Per Serving (1 fillet and 1 cup broccoli): Calories: 155; Total Fat: 4g; Saturated Fat: 1g; Sodium: 710mg; Carbohydrates: 7g; Fiber: 3g; Protein: 23g

Coquilles St. Jacques (Scallops and Mushrooms)

Scallops are nutritious: high in protein, vitamin B$_{12}$, iodine, phosphorus, selenium, choline, and zinc. They have a delicate, mildly sweet flavor and don't need much to make them delicious. Coquilles St. Jacques is a classic dish that will impress any dinner guest or make any occasion more special. **MAKES 4 SERVINGS**

Olive oil cooking spray

2 cups cauliflower purée (see Ingredient Tip)

4 tablespoons nutritional yeast, divided

1 tablespoon chopped fresh parsley

4 teaspoons sherry vinegar

2 teaspoons minced garlic

2 teaspoons chopped fresh chives

3 cups sliced baby portobello mushrooms

1 pound fresh scallops

¼ cup coconut flour

2 teaspoons extra-virgin olive oil

MAKE-AHEAD

Prep time: 15 minutes
Cook time: 45 minutes

Ingredient Tip: With the rise in popularity of cauliflower, it may be possible to find puréed cauliflower in the frozen section of your local grocery store. To make your own, simply steam 3 cups of cauliflower florets until tender (in a pot on the stovetop with ¼ inch of water), drain well, and blend or purée it in a food processor until smooth.

1. Preheat the oven to 350°F. Grease a 9-by-13-inch glass baking dish evenly with cooking spray and set it aside.

2. In a large mixing bowl, combine the cauliflower purée, 2 tablespoons of nutritional yeast, the parsley, sherry vinegar, garlic, and chives. Mix well.

3. Stir in the mushrooms.

4. Gently stir in the scallops until they are well coated.

5. Pour the ingredients into the prepared baking dish and spread out the scallops so they are in a single layer.

6. In a small bowl, mix together the remaining 2 tablespoons of nutritional yeast, the coconut flour, and olive oil until combined. Sprinkle over the scallops.

7. Bake for 45 minutes, or until the crust is golden brown and the scallops reach an internal temperature of 135°F.

   Make-Ahead Tip: For a quick and easy dinner, prepare the dish ahead of time through step 6. Store it in the refrigerator until you are ready to cook, and then resume at step 7.

Per Serving (¼ prepared recipe): Calories: 257; Total Fat: 6g; Saturated Fat: 1g; Sodium: 193mg; Carbohydrates: 22g; Fiber: 11g; Protein: 31g

Crab and Asparagus Casserole

Crab contains many nutrients to support thyroid health, like selenium and omega-3 fatty acids. In this recipe, it's paired with asparagus, an antioxidant-packed vegetable. The flavors in this casserole come together to create a truly decadent meal—rich and creamy, savory and salty. **MAKES 4 SERVINGS**

Olive oil cooking spray

2 cups cauliflower purée (see Ingredient Tip)

2 cups diced asparagus

1 cup cauliflower florets

¼ cup sliced scallions, green and white parts

¼ cup nutritional yeast, divided

2 tablespoons red wine vinegar

1 tablespoon chopped fresh tarragon

1 tablespoon freshly squeezed lemon juice

1 pound crabmeat

2 tablespoons coconut flour

1 teaspoon extra-virgin olive oil

MAKE-AHEAD

Prep time: 5 minutes
Cook time: 45 minutes

Ingredient Tip: With the rise in popularity of cauliflower, it may be possible to find puréed cauliflower in the frozen section of your local grocery store. To make your own, simply steam 3 cups of cauliflower florets until tender (in a pot on the stovetop with ¼ inch of water), drain well, and blend or purée it in a food processor until smooth.

1. Preheat the oven to 350°F. Grease a 9-by-13-inch glass baking dish evenly with the cooking spray and set it aside.

2. In a large mixing bowl, combine the cauliflower purée, asparagus, cauliflower florets, scallions, 3 tablespoons of nutritional yeast, the red wine vinegar, tarragon, and lemon juice. Stir well.

3. Gently stir in the crabmeat.

4. Pour the mixture into the prepared baking dish.

5. In a small bowl, mix together the remaining 1 tablespoon of nutritional yeast, the coconut flour, and olive oil until combined. Sprinkle over the casserole.

6. Bake for 45 minutes, or until the top is golden brown and the casserole reaches an internal temperature of 135°F.

   Make-Ahead Tip: For a quick and easy dinner, prepare the dish through step 5. Store it in the refrigerator until you're ready to cook, and then resume at step 6.

   Variation Tip: Instead of crabmeat, you can substitute flaked white fish like cod or haddock.

Per Serving (¼ prepared recipe): Calories: 257; Total Fat: 5g; Saturated Fat: 1g; Sodium: 449mg; Carbohydrates: 19g; Fiber: 10g; Protein: 37g

Thai Coconut Steamed Mussels

Mussels may not be your traditional everyday food, but they are very nutritious and offer a host of health benefits. Rich in protein, they also contain vitamins, minerals, and the omega-3 fatty acids needed for reducing inflammation. Mussels contain many of the nutrients needed to support optimal thyroid health, including iron, zinc, and B vitamins. This dish is served in a warm, savory broth, so no one will miss the butter. **MAKES 4 SERVINGS**

1 tablespoon
   coconut oil
¼ cup sliced scallions,
   green and white parts
1 tablespoon minced
   fresh gingerroot
1 tablespoon
   minced garlic
1 (15-ounce) can full-fat
   coconut milk

½ teaspoon ground
   turmeric
½ teaspoon salt
Pinch ground cinnamon
Pinch ground cloves
2 tablespoons chopped
   fresh cilantro
2 dozen mussels,
   rinsed and cleaned
   (broken or open ones
   discarded)

**30-MINUTE
ONE-POT**

Prep time: 10 minutes
Cook time: 15 minutes

Ingredient Tip: Many grocery stores carry pre-cleaned frozen mussels in the freezer section. You can also make this dish with clams, another nutritious seafood option.

1. Heat the coconut oil in a 4-quart pot over medium-high heat.

2. When the oil is hot, add the scallions and sauté for 2 minutes.

3. Add the ginger and cook, stirring occasionally, for 1 minute.

4. Add the garlic and cook, stirring frequently, for 1 minute.

5. Add the coconut milk, turmeric, salt, cinnamon, and cloves. Mix well and bring to a boil.

6. Add the cilantro, followed by the mussels.

7. Cover and cook for 10 minutes, or until the mussels have opened. Discard any unopened mussels before serving.

Per Serving (6 mussels): Calories: 318; Total Fat: 30g; Saturated Fat: 26g; Sodium: 416mg; Carbohydrates: 10g; Fiber: 3g; Protein: 8g

Sheet Pan Shrimp and Artichokes

Shrimp, a high-protein shellfish, contains many essential nutrients, including selenium, which helps to support thyroid health. In this dish, it is paired with artichokes and lemon juice for classic French flavor. Artichokes contain significant amounts of dietary fiber and the prebiotic fiber known as inulin. Prebiotics are the important fibers that help feed the beneficial probiotics in the gut.

MAKES 4 SERVINGS

2 tablespoons extra-virgin olive oil

1½ tablespoons minced garlic

1 tablespoon Homemade Vegetable Bone Broth (page 162)

1 tablespoon nutritional yeast

1 teaspoon freshly squeezed lemon juice

1 teaspoon sherry vinegar

1 pound large (21/25-count) peeled and deveined raw shrimp

12 ounces frozen artichoke hearts, thawed, or 1 (15-ounce) can artichoke hearts, drained

30-MINUTE

Prep time: 10 minutes
Cook time: 20 minutes

Ingredient Tip: Look for frozen artichoke hearts in your local grocery market freezer section. Check the ingredients list to ensure that artichokes are the only ingredient included.

1. Preheat the oven to 400°F. Line a baking sheet with aluminum foil and set it aside.

2. In a large bowl, whisk together the olive oil, garlic, broth, nutritional yeast, lemon juice, and vinegar until well combined.

3. Add the shrimp and artichoke hearts and toss until the shrimp are well coated.

4. Transfer to the prepared baking sheet. Bake for 10 to 15 minutes, or until the shrimp are pink and opaque.

Per Serving (¼ prepared recipe): Calories: 230; Total Fat: 9g; Saturated Fat: 1g; Sodium: 336mg; Carbohydrates: 11g; Fiber: 6g; Protein: 28g

Grilled Shrimp with Chimichurri Sauce

Shrimp provides the body with thyroid-supporting selenium and B vitamins. Studies have shown that individuals with Hashimoto's who increased their daily intake of selenium were able to reduce their thyroid antibodies. In this recipe, you'll enjoy shrimp skewered with tasty South American–inspired chimichurri sauce. **MAKES 4 SERVINGS**

1 pound large (21/25-count) peeled and deveined raw shrimp

4 (10-inch) metal skewers (or wooden skewers soaked in water for 30 minutes)

½ cup Chimichurri Sauce (page 167), divided

5-INGREDIENT
30-MINUTE

Prep time: 10 minutes
Cook time: 5 minutes

Serving Tip: You can use this method to grill shrimp for convenient meal prep for the upcoming week. Add grilled shrimp to salads and wraps, and keep them stocked for quick and easy dinners.

1. Preheat the grill on high heat.

2. Thread 5 shrimp onto each skewer. Aim to skewer each shrimp through both the tail and the body, creating a C shape to ensure that the shrimp cook evenly and don't fall off.

3. Brush half the chimichurri sauce over the skewered shrimp; set the rest of the sauce aside.

4. Carefully lay the skewers on the grill. Cook for 2 to 3 minutes on one side, then flip them and grill on the other side for 1 to 2 minutes, or until the shrimp is pink and opaque. Remove the skewers from the grill.

5. Pour the remaining chimichurri sauce over the cooked shrimp just before serving.

Per Serving (1 skewer): Calories: 120; Total Fat: 1g; Saturated Fat: 0g; Sodium: 387mg; Carbohydrates: 2g; Fiber: 0g; Protein: 24g

One-Pot Shrimp Bisque

Enjoy restaurant-quality food in the comfort of your home, with no additives or undisclosed ingredients. This soup is made with only high-quality seafood and immune-boosting ingredients like fresh ginger, a rhizome with potent health benefits including strong antioxidant and anti-inflammatory properties.

MAKES 4 SERVINGS

1 tablespoon extra-virgin olive oil

1 cup diced white onion

1 cup diced carrot

½ cup diced celery

½ teaspoon salt

½ pound peeled and deveined raw shrimp, roughly chopped

2 tablespoons minced garlic

3 tablespoons minced fresh gingerroot

1 cup Homemade Vegetable Bone Broth (page 162)

⅛ teaspoon ground cinnamon

2 (15-ounce) cans full-fat coconut milk, shaken

¼ cup chopped fresh cilantro

ONE-POT

Prep time: 10 minutes
Cook time: 45 minutes

Recipe Tip: If you don't have an immersion blender, you can use a traditional blender and blend until smooth. (Just be careful—hot contents can spatter. To prevent this, cover the blender lid with a towel.) Additionally, you could skip this step altogether and enjoy a chunky-style soup.

Cooking Tip: "Sweating" means to lightly cook without browning. You want to remove some of the moisture from the ingredient, but not cook it fully. This is achieved by stirring very frequently.

1. Heat the olive oil in a medium soup pot over medium-high heat.

2. When the oil is hot, add the onion, carrot, celery, and salt. Reduce the heat to medium-low and sweat the vegetables, stirring frequently, until soft, about 10 minutes.

3. Add the shrimp and cook for 2 minutes, or until just opaque.

4. Add the garlic and ginger, and cook for 1 minute.
5. Add the broth and cook for 5 minutes, or until the liquid has reduced by half.
6. Stir in the cinnamon and coconut milk.
7. Increase the heat to medium-high and bring the liquid to a boil. Add the cilantro, reduce the heat to low, cover the pot, and let it simmer for 30 minutes.
8. Using an immersion blender, blend the soup until it becomes a smooth bisque.

Per Serving (1 cup): Calories: 535; Total Fat: 46g; Saturated Fat: 38g; Sodium: 477mg; Carbohydrates: 20g; Fiber: 6g; Protein: 17g

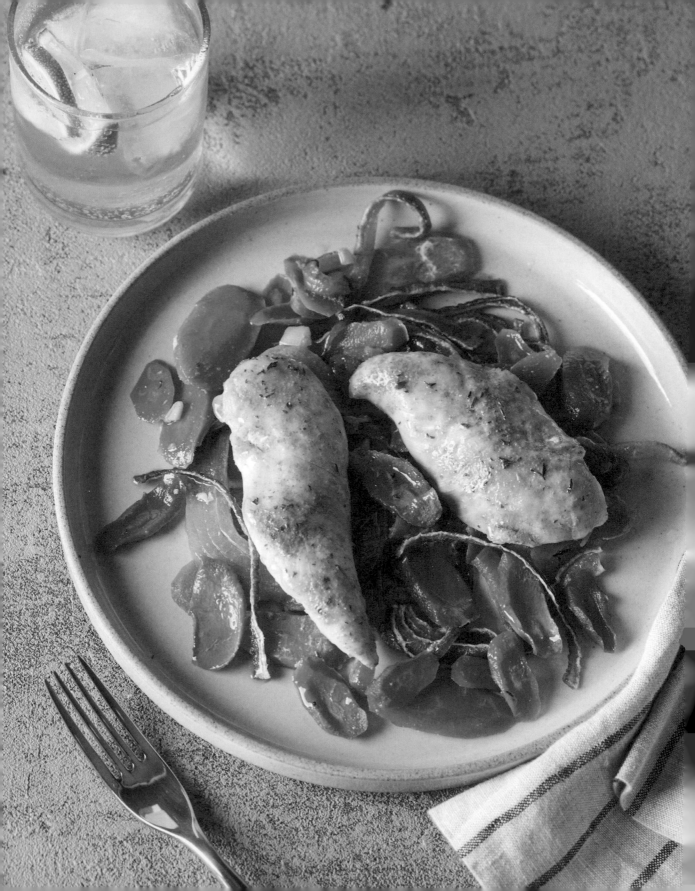

6 *Poultry Mains*

Lemon Spinach Turkey Soup

Making a big batch of soup over the weekend is a great way to secure easy lunch meals for the entire week. This light and delicious soup pairs the fresh flavors of lemon and spinach for a tasty bowl that's great with soups and sandwiches. Spinach is packed with vitamins C and K, folic acid, iron, and calcium, as well as essential B vitamins. **MAKES 8 SERVINGS**

2 tablespoons
  extra-virgin olive oil
2 pounds boneless,
  skinless turkey breast,
  cut into 1-inch cubes
1 cup diced
  yellow onion
1 teaspoon salt, divided
2 cups diced celery
1 cup diced carrots
1 tablespoon
  minced garlic

6 cups Homemade
  Vegetable Bone Broth
  (page 162)
1 bay leaf
2 teaspoons chopped
  fresh thyme
1 teaspoon lemon zest
12 ounces baby spinach
¼ cup freshly squeezed
  lemon juice

**MAKE-AHEAD
ONE-POT**

Prep time: 15 minutes
Cook time: 2 hours
  15 minutes

Make-Ahead Tip: This recipe will make 8 servings, so freeze half if you can't eat it all within a few days.

1. Heat the olive oil in a large soup pot over medium-high heat.

2. When the oil is hot, add the cubed turkey and cook for 5 to 10 minutes, or until the turkey begins to brown.

3. Add the onion and ½ teaspoon of salt and cook, stirring occasionally, for 2 to 3 minutes, or until the onion begins to turn translucent.

4. Add the celery and remaining ½ teaspoon of salt and cook, stirring occasionally, for 2 to 3 minutes.

5. Add the carrots and cook, stirring occasionally, for another 2 to 3 minutes.

6. Add the garlic and cook, stirring frequently, for 1 to 2 minutes.

7. Add the broth, bay leaf, thyme, and lemon zest. Increase the heat to high and bring to a boil.

8. Once the soup is boiling, reduce the heat to a simmer, cover with a tight-fitting lid, and cook for 2 hours, stirring occasionally.

9. After 2 hours, increase the heat to high, return the soup to a boil, and then reduce the heat to low and stir in the spinach and lemon juice. Let the soup simmer for another 15 minutes to wilt the spinach and marry all the flavors. Serve hot.

Per Serving (1 cup): Calories: 210; Total Fat: 6g; Saturated Fat: 1g; Sodium: 494mg; Carbohydrates: 10g; Fiber: 3g; Protein: 29g

One-Pot Zuppa Toscana

Zuppa Toscana, or Tuscan soup, is comfort food in a bowl, even for those follow- ing the AIP. It's packed with health-supportive ingredients, including kale, which adds a pop of color and a load of nutrition. In fact, kale has been named one of the most nutrient-dense foods on the planet thanks to its incredible vitamin and mineral content. A single cup of raw kale contains more than twice the rec- ommended daily value of vitamin A and more than six times the recommended daily value of vitamin K. **MAKES 4 SERVINGS**

1 tablespoon
   extra-virgin olive oil
1 pound ground
   chicken or pork
1 tablespoon
   minced garlic
1 medium sweet
   onion, diced
1 teaspoon AIP Spice
   Blend (page 160)

6 cups Homemade
   Vegetable Bone Broth
   (page 162)
3 cups diced sweet
   potatoes
6 cups baby
   kale, packed
1 cup coconut milk
2 tablespoons
   coconut cream

**30-MINUTE
ONE-POT**

Prep time: 5 minutes
Cook time: 25 minutes

Substitution Tip: You can use any type of ground meat in this recipe, includ- ing chicken, turkey, or pork. You can swap the kale for spinach, too.

1. In a large stock pot over medium heat, combine the olive oil and ground meat.

2. Cook for 5 minutes, stirring frequently, until the meat is browned. Drain the excess fat if desired.

3. Add the garlic, onion and spice blend. Cook, stirring occasionally, until the onion starts to become translucent, 3 to 5 minutes.

4. Add the broth and sweet potatoes, increase the heat to medium-high, and bring to a boil.

5. Boil for 2 minutes, then reduce the heat to low. Cover and simmer for 15 minutes.

6. Stir in the kale until wilted. Add the coconut milk and coconut cream, and stir until warmed through. Serve immediately.

Per Serving (¼ prepared recipe): Calories: 591; Total Fat: 32g; Saturated Fat: 20g; Sodium: 354mg; Carbohydrates: 54g; Fiber: 7g; Protein: 27g

Chicken Bacon Ranch Salad

Many people enjoy a hearty salad as an entrée, and this salad does not disappoint. Packed with heart-healthy fats and nutrients from the avocado and great flavor from the bacon and shredded chicken, this meal is low-carb, high-fat, and sure to please your taste buds. One of the only fruits with a high fat content, avocados contain monounsaturated fatty acids, which are associated with reducing inflammation in the body. **MAKES 4 SERVINGS**

6 cups roughly chopped
    Boston Bibb lettuce
1 pound Slow Cooker
    Shredded Chicken
    (page 107)

4 slices cooked uncured
    bacon, crumbled
2 avocados, pitted,
    scooped, and diced
½ cup Creamy Ranch
    Dressing (page 172)

**5-INGREDIENT
30-MINUTE**

Prep time: 10 minutes

1. Divide the lettuce among 4 bowls.
2. Evenly distribute the shredded chicken, bacon, and avocados among the bowls.
3. Just before serving, top with the dressing.

Per Serving (1 salad): Calories: 456; Total Fat: 33g; Saturated Fat: 17g; Sodium: 534mg; Carbohydrates: 14g; Fiber: 7g; Protein: 32g

Ingredient Tip: You can also simply use diced cooked chicken breast. Use any of your favorite lettuces, like iceberg, romaine, or mixed greens. Alternatively, skip the salad greens and combine the rest of the ingredients to use as a filling for lettuce wraps, cucumber bites, or Grain-Free Tortillas (page 174).

Rainbow Chicken Salad

The old saying "eat the rainbow" has truth: A healthy diet is full of a variety of foods. The different colors in whole, all-natural foods are indicators of different nutrients. This rainbow salad features antioxidant health benefits from kale, red cabbage, and carrots for a detoxifying, high-fiber meal that is pretty to look at and deliciously satisfying to eat. **MAKES 4 SERVINGS**

2 cups chopped
  kale leaves
2 cups chopped
  red cabbage
2 cups matchstick-cut
  carrots
½ cup chopped fresh
  cilantro
½ cup chopped
  fresh parsley
¼ cup sliced scallions,
  green and white parts

2 avocados, pitted,
  scooped, and diced
1 cup Slow Cooker
  Shredded Chicken
  (page 107)
½ cup Green Goddess
  Dressing (page 171)
½ cup pomegranate
  arils (optional; see
  Ingredient Tip)

30-MINUTE
MAKE-AHEAD
ONE-BOWL

Prep time: 20 minutes

1. In a large bowl, toss together the kale, cabbage, carrots, cilantro, parsley, and scallions. Divide among 4 smaller bowls or meal prep containers.

2. Top each salad evenly with the diced avocado and shredded chicken.

3. Just before serving, top each with the dressing and pomegranate arils (if using).

Per Serving (1 salad): Calories: 367; Total Fat: 22g; Saturated Fat: 3g; Sodium: 252mg; Carbohydrates: 21g; Fiber: 9g; Protein: 26g

Make-Ahead Tip: If making this in advance, wait to cut the avocado until just ready to serve, as it will brown quickly. Top with the dressing and pomegranate arils right before serving.

Ingredient Tip: Pomegranate arils add a delicious pop of color and flavor to this salad, but they are hard to find at certain times of the year. If you do not have fresh pomegranate available, simply omit this optional ingredient.

Substitution Tip: If you don't have Slow Cooker Shredded Chicken (page 107) prepared, simply used diced cooked chicken breast.

Grape Chicken Salad Wraps

Many people following an AIP diet find themselves missing traditional mayo-based salads such as chicken salad or tuna salad. Luckily, you can create your own rich and flavorful mayo substitute using creamy avocado. Feel free to customize this recipe to whatever ways you traditionally prepare chicken salad, using ingredients that are approved on your current diet. **MAKES 4 SERVINGS**

1 cup Slow Cooker Shredded Chicken (page 107)

½ cup quartered red grapes

½ cup finely diced celery

¼ cup finely diced red onion

½ avocado, pitted, scooped, and diced

2 tablespoons coconut cream, at room temperature

½ teaspoon AIP Spice Blend (page 160)

4 Grain-Free Tortillas (page 174) or lettuce leaves, for serving

30-MINUTE
ONE-BOWL

Prep time: 10 minutes

Ingredient Tip: If you do not have Slow Cooker Shredded Chicken (page 107) prepared, simply used diced cooked chicken breast.

1. In a medium bowl, combine the shredded chicken, grapes, celery, and red onion.

2. Mix in the avocado, coconut cream, and spice blend. Stir until well combined.

3. Serve wrapped in the tortillas or lettuce leaves.

Per Serving (½ cup salad; 1 wrap): Calories: 262; Total Fat: 10g; Saturated Fat: 3g; Sodium: 312mg; Carbohydrates: 19g; Fiber: 4g; Protein: 23g

Lemon Basil Chicken Sliders

These juicy mini burgers are bursting with the flavors delivered by fresh basil, parsley, and oregano. Basil is a powerful antioxidant, anti-inflammatory herb with a bright flavor that adds important nutrients to this meal. Studies have shown that this herb also contains antibacterial properties, acts as a natural adaptogen in the body, and may even help fight cancer. **MAKES 8 SLIDERS**

1 small zucchini, roughly chopped

½ small red onion, roughly chopped

3 garlic cloves

¼ cup fresh basil leaves, packed

2 tablespoons fresh parsley leaves, packed

1 teaspoon fresh oregano leaves, packed

1 pound ground chicken

2 tablespoons freshly squeezed lemon juice

1 tablespoon coconut liquid aminos

¼ teaspoon salt

1 tablespoon coconut oil

30-MINUTE

Prep time: 15 minutes
Cook time: 10 minutes

Substitution Tip: You can use ground chicken or ground turkey interchangeably in this recipe. Alternatively, shape the ground meat mixture into smaller, round balls to make meatballs.

Serving Tip: Enjoy these sliders in a salad, paired with Baked Rutabaga French Fries (page 57), or topped with Quick Pickled Red Onions (page 48) and Creamy Coconut Milk Yogurt (page 177).

1. In a food processor, pulse the zucchini, onion, garlic, basil, parsley, and oregano until finely minced.

2. In a large bowl, combine the zucchini mixture, ground chicken, lemon juice, coconut aminos, and salt until well combined.

3. Shape the mixture into 8 evenly sized patties. Set aside.

4. In a large cast-iron skillet, heat the coconut oil over medium-low heat. Add the burgers and cook for 5 minutes per side, or until they reach an internal temperature of 165°F. Serve immediately.

Per Serving (2 [2-ounce] burger patties): Calories: 184; Total Fat: 9g; Saturated Fat: 3g; Sodium: 332mg; Carbohydrates: 5g; Fiber: 1g; Protein: 20g

Mediterranean Chicken Pizzas

Enjoying your favorite foods is not impossible on the autoimmune protocol—it just takes a bit of preparation and creativity. Many of the ingredients used to make this pizza are from chapter 9 (page 159), so you may already have a few prepared ahead of time, making it easier to throw this recipe together on a Friday night. **MAKES 4 SERVINGS**

½ cup Creamy Coconut Milk Yogurt (page 177)

1 tablespoon minced garlic

1 teaspoon AIP Spice Blend (page 160)

4 AIP-Friendly Flatbreads (page 176)

1 cup chopped spinach

½ cup Garlic Olive Tapenade (page 173)

1 cup Slow Cooker Shredded Chicken (page 107) or diced cooked chicken breast

2 cups baby arugula

1 teaspoon extra-virgin olive oil

1 teaspoon balsamic vinegar

¼ teaspoon salt

30-MINUTE

Prep time: 10 minutes
Cook time: 15 minutes

Ingredient Tip: Use this recipe as a base for any type of pizza you want to make. Just ensure that all of your pizza toppings are AIP-friendly, and you can enjoy this classic comfort food again and again.

1. Preheat the oven to 350°F.
2. In a small bowl, mix together the coconut milk yogurt, minced garlic, and spice blend.

3. Place the flatbreads on a baking sheet. Spread a thin layer of the yogurt mixture over each flatbread.

4. Top each with the chopped spinach, tapenade, and shredded chicken.

5. Bake for 15 minutes, or until the edges are browned and everything is heated through.

6. Meanwhile, gently toss the arugula with the olive oil, balsamic vinegar, and salt.

7. Remove the pizzas from the oven and top them with the arugula mixture. Slice and serve immediately.

Per Serving (1 pizza): Calories: 423; Total Fat: 26g; Saturated Fat: 14g; Sodium: 1,167mg; Carbohydrates: 24g; Fiber: 9g; Protein: 27g

Chimichurri Baked Chicken Wings

Chicken wings get a bad rap because they are traditionally fried in oil, but baking is an excellent way to enjoy this classic party food staple. This lean protein contains calcium, iron, magnesium, and phosphorus. You can make these skin on or skin off and swap in any other sauce of your choice. **MAKES 4 SERVINGS**

Olive oil cooking spray
1 pound chicken wings
  (skin on or off)

1 cup Chimichurri Sauce
  (page 167), plus more
  for serving

5-INGREDIENT
30-MINUTE

Prep time: 5 minutes
Cook time: 25 minutes

1. Preheat the oven to 425°F. Line a baking sheet with aluminum foil and spray with cooking spray. Set aside.

2. In a large bowl, toss together the chicken wings and sauce until well coated.

3. Spread the chicken wings evenly on the baking sheet. Bake for 25 minutes, or until the wings reach an internal temperature of 165°F.

4. Serve with additional sauce as desired.

Serving Tip: Try this recipe with Sweet Beet Vinaigrette (page 169) or Apple Cider Vinaigrette (page 170) for a different flavor combination.

Per Serving (4 ounces chicken, skin off): Calories: 271; Total Fat: 18g; Saturated Fat: 5g; Sodium: 453mg; Carbohydrates: 4g; Fiber: 0g; Protein: 21g

Chicken Egg Roll in a Bowl

Takeout options are typically limited for those following the autoimmune protocol, since it's difficult to know what is actually in the food. Thankfully, you can still enjoy the flavors of Chinese takeout egg rolls with this recipe, which is served in a bowl instead of a wrapper. Before starting, ensure that all your ingredients are prepped and ready to go, as the stir-fry cooking process is very fast-paced.

MAKES 4 SERVINGS

2 tablespoons
extra-virgin olive oil

1 pound ground chicken

½ cup sliced scallions,
green and white parts

2 cups shredded
green cabbage

1 cup shredded
red cabbage

2 cups shredded carrots

2 teaspoons minced
peeled fresh
gingerroot

4 cups shredded
Napa cabbage

12 ounces Homemade
Stir-Fry Sauce
(page 165)

**30-MINUTE
ONE-POT**

Prep time: 20 minutes
Cook time: 10 minutes

Ingredient Tip: To make the preparation of this dish easier, swap the Napa cabbage, green cabbage, and red cabbage for 2 (16-ounce) bags of pre-cut coleslaw mix. This can be purchased in most grocery stores. Just read the ingredients list to be sure that cabbage and carrots are the only ingredients listed.

Serving Tip: Enjoy this dish as is or served over From-Scratch Cauliflower Rice (page 60) for a hearty twist.

1. Heat a large skillet or wok over medium-high heat. Once the pan is hot, add the olive oil and ground chicken and stir-fry for 2 minutes, or until the chicken is browned.

2. Move the chicken to the outside perimeter of the skillet and increase the heat to high.

3. Add the scallions to the center of the skillet and cook for 1 minute, stirring only the scallions (not the chicken), until they are slightly tender. Move the cooked scallions to the outer edge of the skillet with the chicken.

continued

4. Add the green cabbage to the center of the skillet, stir for 1 minute until the cabbage is slightly tender, and then move it to the outer edge of the skillet.

5. Repeat the stir-frying process with the red cabbage, then the carrots, and then the ginger.

6. When the ginger starts to get fragrant, add the Napa cabbage on top of it.

7. When the Napa cabbage is slightly tender, after about 1 minute, push all the ingredients from the edge of the skillet to the center and stir everything together.

8. Add the stir-fry sauce and continue to stir for 2 minutes. When the sauce has reduced by half, remove the skillet from the heat, scoop the stir-fry into bowls, and serve.

Per Serving (¼ prepared recipe): Calories: 314; Total Fat: 16g; Saturated Fat: 4g; Sodium: 157mg; Carbohydrates: 21g; Fiber: 5g; Protein: 22g

Slow Cooker Shredded Chicken

Having a go-to recipe like this is great if you are cooking in bulk to prepare for the week or to stock the freezer. The cooked chicken can be used for salads, tacos, wraps, sandwiches, and more. Chicken contains many essential amino acids, high-quality protein, and nutrients like selenium, which is crucial for thyroid health. **MAKES 4 SERVINGS**

2 pounds boneless, skinless chicken thighs

1 tablespoon AIP Spice Blend (page 160)

½ cup Homemade Vegetable Bone Broth (page 162)

1 teaspoon apple cider vinegar

5-INGREDIENT
MAKE-AHEAD
ONE-POT

Prep time: 5 minutes
Cook time: 3 hours

1. Place the chicken thighs in a slow cooker and sprinkle with the spice blend.

2. Pour in the broth and vinegar.

3. Cook on high for 3 hours, or until the chicken falls apart easily when poked with a fork.

4. Using two forks, shred the chicken. Serve immediately, or portion the shredded chicken and liquid into airtight containers and refrigerate or freeze them for easy meals throughout the week. If frozen, thaw the container in the refrigerator overnight before warming. If refrigerated, serve cold or hot.

Serving Tip: Try this chicken with the Chicken Bacon Ranch Salad (page 98).

Make-Ahead Tip: You can easily double this recipe for make-ahead meal prep if you have a 6-quart or larger slow cooker.

Per Serving (½ cup): Calories: 261; Total Fat: 9g; Saturated Fat: 2g; Sodium: 260mg; Carbohydrates: 0g; Fiber: 0g; Protein: 44g

AIP-Friendly Fried Chicken

Chicken drumsticks are a delicious staple food for many households, especially during the summer months. Eating fried foods is not ideal on the AIP, but a protocol-friendly recipe like this can be helpful when entertaining or bringing a dish to a social event. Chicken contains essential amino acids, high-quality protein, and important nutrients like selenium, making this recipe both nutritious and delicious. **MAKES 4 SERVINGS**

1 cup coconut milk
¼ teaspoon freshly
   squeezed lemon juice
1½ pounds chicken
   drumsticks (about 8)
1 cup cassava flour

2½ tablespoons
   AIP Spice Blend
   (page 160)
2 cups melted coconut
   oil, plus more
   as needed

30-MINUTE

Prep time: 10 minutes
Cook time: 20 minutes

Substitution Tip: You can use this same process to fry other cuts of meat, including turkey drumsticks or bone-in chicken thighs.

1. In a large bowl, whisk together the coconut milk and lemon juice. Place the chicken drumsticks in the coconut milk mixture and set aside.

2. In a medium bowl, whisk together the cassava flour and spice blend.

3. Remove the chicken drumsticks from the coconut milk, shake off the excess liquid, and place them in the bowl with the flour. Roll until each drumstick is well coated. Set aside.

4. Fill a large skillet one-third full with melted coconut oil. Place the skillet over medium heat and, using a digital instant-read thermometer, bring the oil temperature to 325°F.

5. Carefully place the chicken drumsticks in the hot oil and turn the heat to high until the oil returns to 325°F. Reduce the heat once the temperature is reached, and work to keep the temperature as consistent as possible. Cook the chicken on one side for 5 minutes.

6. After 5 minutes, flip the chicken and cook for an additional 5 minutes.

7. Flip the chicken one more time and allow it to cook for another 5 minutes, or until it reaches an internal temperature of 165°F.

8. Transfer the cooked chicken pieces to a wire rack lined with paper towels to absorb excess oil. Serve immediately.

Per Serving (2 drumsticks): Calories: 525; Total Fat: 34g; Saturated Fat: 19g; Sodium: 941mg; Carbohydrates: 29g; Fiber: 5g; Protein: 29g

Creamy Chicken Florentine

Chicken Florentine is a classic Italian comfort food dish that the whole family will enjoy. Golden-brown chicken breasts are topped with a creamy sauce and served over a bed of spinach. Studies have shown that eating a diet rich in leafy greens like spinach can offer numerous health benefits, including protecting against cognitive decline or "brain fog" that often plagues those with Hashimoto's. **MAKES 4 SERVINGS**

1 pound boneless, skinless chicken breast, cut into 4 equal-size pieces and pounded thin
½ cup cassava flour
1 tablespoon coconut oil
¼ cup sliced scallions, green and white parts

6 ounces baby spinach
¼ teaspoon salt
3 tablespoons Homemade Vegetable Bone Broth (page 162), divided
1½ cups Cauliflower Alfredo Sauce (page 166)

30-MINUTE

Prep time: 20 minutes
Cook time: 10 minutes

Serving Tip: Serve this dish inside Roasted Spaghetti Squash Bowls (page 66) for the ultimate comfort meal.

1. In a shallow bowl, dust the chicken breast in the cassava flour until well coated.

2. In a large skillet over medium heat, melt the coconut oil.

3. When the oil is hot, carefully add the coated chicken breasts and cook for 2 to 3 minutes on one side.

4. Flip the chicken and cook for another 2 to 3 minutes, or until the chicken is opaque throughout. Move the cooked chicken breasts to the outside edges of the pan.

5. Add the scallions to the center of the pan and sauté for 2 minutes.

6. Add the spinach, salt, and 1 tablespoon of broth to the center of the pan, and stir constantly until the spinach is wilted.

7. Divide the spinach among 4 plates and top each serving with a piece of chicken.

8. Add the Alfredo sauce and remaining 2 tablespoons of broth to the pan, and stir for 1 minute to combine and heat the sauce.

9. Spoon the sauce over the chicken and serve immediately.

Per Serving (¼ prepared recipe): Calories: 245; Total Fat: 8g; Saturated Fat: 3g; Sodium: 475mg; Carbohydrates: 17g; Fiber: 5g; Protein: 29g

One-Pot Whole Roasted Chicken

Knowing how to cook a whole roasted chicken in one pot is a priceless kitchen trick, and it's easier than you may think. This dish is perfect for enjoying with the family over the weekend, for Sunday supper, or for advance meal prepping. Cooking the whole bird locks in the optimal nutritional benefits, since animal bones are a rich source of collagen, amino acids like proline and glycine, and important minerals. **MAKES 8 SERVINGS**

2 tablespoons
    extra-virgin olive oil
1 tablespoon AIP Spice
    Blend (page 160)
1 whole chicken (about
    4 pounds)

1 cup diced white onion
1 cup diced celery
1 cup diced carrots
1 cup Homemade
    Vegetable Bone Broth
    (page 162)

**MAKE-AHEAD
ONE-POT**

Prep time: 10 minutes
Cook time: 1 hour
    10 minutes

1. Preheat the oven to 400°F.
2. In a small bowl, mix together the olive oil and spice blend. Generously rub this mixture all over the chicken.
3. In a Dutch oven, combine the onion, celery, and carrots. Set the chicken on top of the vegetables, and pour the broth over the chicken. Bake for 1 hour, or until the chicken reaches an internal temperature of 160°F.
4. Remove the chicken from the oven and allow the meat to rest, covered, for 10 minutes, or until the internal temperature rises to 165°F.
5. Carve the chicken just before serving.

Make-Ahead Tip: Save the chicken carcass after you have removed all of the meat—this is the perfect base for bone broth (page 162). If using this recipe for meal prep, carve the chicken and separate out the breasts, thighs, drumsticks, and wings.

Per Serving (4 ounces chicken): Calories: 287; Total Fat: 22g; Saturated Fat: 6g; Sodium: 160mg; Carbohydrates: 4g; Fiber: 1g; Protein: 19g

Sheet Pan Turmeric Chicken and Carrots

Most widely known for their vitamin A content, carrots are an antioxidant-rich root vegetable with a vibrant orange color, thanks to their high concentration of beta-carotene. Carrots have been a dietary staple in many cultures for hundreds of years. Enjoy their benefits in this delicious, healthy baking sheet supper.

MAKES 4 SERVINGS

1 tablespoon extra-virgin olive oil

1 tablespoon raw honey

1 pound boneless, skinless chicken tenderloins

1 red onion, sliced

4 carrots, peeled and thinly sliced on a bias

¼ teaspoon ground turmeric

¼ teaspoon AIP Spice Blend (page 160)

½ teaspoon kosher salt

30-MINUTE
ONE-PAN

Prep time: 10 minutes
Cook time: 20 minutes

Serving Tip: Serve with From-Scratch Cauliflower Rice (page 60) or Baked Rutabaga French Fries (page 57).

1. Preheat the oven to 350°F. Line a baking sheet with aluminum foil; set aside.

2. In a small bowl, whisk together the olive oil and honey. Set aside.

3. Place the chicken, red onion, and sliced carrots on the prepared baking sheet.

4. Sprinkle the turmeric, spice blend, and salt over the chicken and vegetables.

5. Drizzle with the olive oil mixture.

6. Bake for 20 minutes, or until the chicken reaches an internal temperature of 165°F.

Per Serving (½ cup): Calories: 202; Total Fat: 5g; Saturated Fat: 1g; Sodium: 409mg; Carbohydrates: 13g; Fiber: 2g; Protein: 27g

Maple and Bacon Roasted Turkey Breast

Many people worry that when they start the AIP, they won't be able to enjoy social eating experiences. Fortunately, this dish will please everyone, regardless of whether they are following the AIP or not. This dish is so good, you will be proud to serve it as you entertain, and no one will even have to know that they're adhering to your protocol. **MAKES 8 SERVINGS**

1 pound sweet potatoes, peeled and cut into 3-inch-thick rounds
¼ cup Homemade Vegetable Bone Broth (page 162)
2 pounds split bone-in turkey breast
½ teaspoon kosher salt
3 tablespoons pure maple syrup
6 slices thick-cut uncured bacon

**5-INGREDIENT
MAKE-AHEAD
ONE-POT**

Prep time: 10 minutes
Cook time: 2 hours

Make-Ahead Tip: You will likely have leftovers from this dish. Pack them in individual containers for ready-prepped meals throughout the week.

1. Preheat the oven to 325°F.
2. Arrange the sweet potatoes around the edges of a Dutch oven. Gently pour in the broth.
3. Place the turkey breast in the center of the Dutch oven with the sweet potatoes surrounding it.

4. Season with the salt and maple syrup.

5. Lay the bacon slices over the turkey, covering the breast as much as possible. Try to tuck the ends of the bacon slices under the turkey.

6. Transfer the pot to the oven and roast the turkey for 1 hour 45 minutes to 2 hours, or until it reaches an internal temperature of 160°F. Remove the pot from the oven and allow the meat to rest until it reaches an internal temperature of 165°F.

7. Carve the turkey breast and serve with the sweet potatoes.

Ingredient Tip: You can also use a boneless turkey breast for this recipe, but bone-in provides more flavor and collagen, an important nutrient for gut health.

Per Serving (⅛ prepared recipe): Calories: 311; Total Fat: 12g; Saturated Fat: 4g; Sodium: 522mg; Carbohydrates: 17g; Fiber: 2g; Protein: 29g

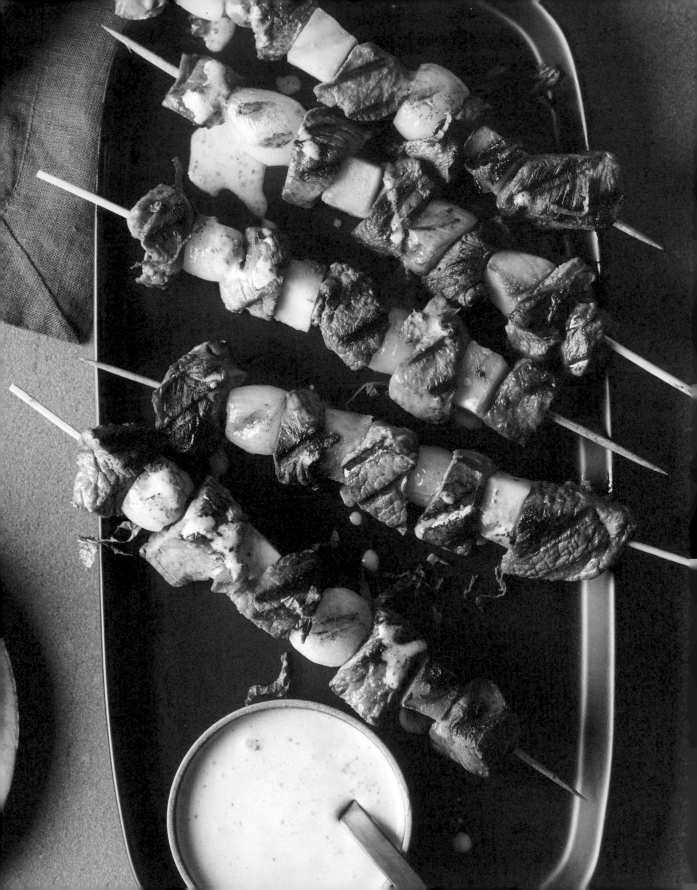

7 Beef, Lamb, and Pork Mains

Dutch Oven Pork with Apples and Fennel

This easy one-pan meal will fill your home with the sweet scent of apples and fennel baking together. Pork tenderloin is considered a lean pork option, providing less fat and fewer calories per ounce than other cuts. Pork is a good source of the mineral selenium, which helps control the activity of thyroid hormones in the body. **MAKES 4 SERVINGS**

4 Granny Smith apples, cored and sliced ¼ inch thick

1 fennel bulb, sliced ¼ inch thick

1 pound pork tenderloin

¼ teaspoon salt

1 tablespoon extra-virgin olive oil

Chopped fennel fronds, for garnish

**5-INGREDIENT
ONE-PAN**

Prep time: 10 minutes
Cook time: 45 minutes
Rest time: 10 minutes

1. Preheat the oven to 350°F.

2. Arrange the sliced apples and fennel in the bottom of a Dutch oven or roasting pan.

3. Lay the pork tenderloin on top of the apples and fennel. Sprinkle the pork with the salt and drizzle with the olive oil.

4. Cover with a tight-fitting lid or aluminum foil and bake for about 45 minutes, or until the pork reaches an internal temperature of 140°F.

5. Remove the pot from the oven and allow the meat to rest, covered, for 5 to 10 minutes, or until the internal temperature reaches 145°F.

6. Slice the pork and serve with the cooked apples and fennel, sprinkled with chopped fennel fronds.

Cooking Tip: A digital instant-read thermometer with an alarm is ideal for cooking cuts of meat such as pork tenderloin. It allows for greater control over the cooking process, and it ensures that you do not overcook the meat.

Serving Tip: You can enjoy this meal as is or served over Garlic Mashed Rutabagas (page 69).

Per Serving (4 ounces): Calories: 266; Total Fat: 7g; Saturated Fat: 2g; Sodium: 449mg; Carbohydrates: 31g; Fiber: 5g; Protein: 22g

Roast Pork with Sauerkraut and Rutabagas

For some families, pork and sauerkraut may be a familiar comfort food. Sauerkraut, also known as fermented cabbage, has earned its stature in the world of gut health because of its prebiotic and probiotic health benefits. The fermentation process creates important probiotics, which have been shown to be beneficial to digestive and immune health. Check the ingredient labels to ensure that cabbage, water, and salt are the only ingredients used, and enjoy it in moderation because of its potentially high iodine content. **MAKES 4 SERVINGS**

4 cups peeled and diced rutabagas

1 pound pork tenderloin

1 teaspoon AIP Spice Blend (page 160)

½ teaspoon kosher salt

2 cups sauerkraut

½ cup Homemade Vegetable Bone Broth (page 162)

**5-INGREDIENT
ONE-POT**

Prep time: 10 minutes
Cook time: 3 hours

Ingredient Tip: You can substitute any AIP-friendly root vegetable for the rutabaga in this dish, such as turnips, carrots, or parsnips.

1. Place the diced rutabagas in a slow cooker. Lay the pork tenderloin on top of the rutabagas and sprinkle with the spice blend and salt.

2. Top the pork and rutabagas with the sauerkraut, and pour in the broth.

3. Cover and cook on high for 3 hours, or until the pork reaches an internal temperature of 145°F.

Per Serving (¼ prepared recipe): Calories: 184; Total Fat: 4g; Saturated Fat: 1g; Sodium: 1088mg; Carbohydrates: 14g; Fiber: 6g; Protein: 23g

Bok Choy Pork Stir-Fry

Baby bok choy is a dark leafy green vegetable commonly found in the Asian section of most grocery stores, typically near the fresh ginger. This staple in Chinese and South Asian cuisine is a tender, mild-flavored member of the cabbage family that cooks quickly. Bok choy is an excellent source of dietary fiber and vitamins like A, C, and K. **MAKES 4 SERVINGS**

1 pound pork
 tenderloin
2 tablespoons
 cassava flour
2 tablespoons
 extra-virgin olive oil
1 cup thinly sliced
 white onion

2 cups sliced
 mushrooms
1 pound baby bok choy,
 sliced lengthwise into
 ½-inch slices
12 ounces Homemade
 Stir-Fry Sauce
 (page 165)

30-MINUTE

Prep time: 20 minutes
Cook time: 10 minutes

Substitution Tip: You can easily substitute the pork tenderloin with chicken tenderloin. If you cannot find baby bok choy in the grocery store, opt for mature bok choy or another dark green leafy vegetable like spinach, kale, collard greens, or mustard greens.

Serving Tip: Enjoy this dish as is or served over From-Scratch Cauliflower Rice (page 60).

1. Cut the pork tenderloin in half lengthwise, and cut each half on the bias into ¼-inch-thick slices.

2. Place the pork slices into a large bowl, add the cassava flour, and toss until coated.

3. Heat a large skillet or wok over medium-high heat. When the pan is hot, add the extra-virgin olive oil.

4. Add the pork to the pan, laying all the pieces flat. Brown on one side for 1 minute, then flip each piece and brown the second side for 1 minute.

5. Move the pork to the outer edges of the pan. Increase the heat to high, and add the onion to the center of the pan, continuously stirring just the onion for 2 minutes.

6. When the onion is slightly tender, move it to the outer edges of the pan with the pork. Add the mushrooms to the center of the pan, and stir them continuously for 1 minute. When the mushrooms are tender, move them to the outer edges with the pork and onion.

7. Add the bok choy to the center of the pan and stir it continuously for 1 minute. When the bok choy is slightly tender, start mixing in all the other ingredients from the outside edges of the pan.

8. Add the stir-fry sauce and mix everything together. Continue to cook for 2 minutes, or until the sauce reduces by half and starts to thicken.

Per Serving (¼ prepared recipe): Calories: 248; Total Fat: 11g; Saturated Fat: 2g; Sodium: 402mg; Carbohydrates: 13g; Fiber: 2g; Protein: 24g

Pork Tapenade Roulade

A roulade is a traditional dish typically made by topping a flat piece of meat with a soft filling and rolling it up into a spiral. It is a bit time-consuming to prepare, but the final presentation of this dish makes it perfect for any special occasion.

MAKES 4 SERVINGS

1 pound pork tenderloin

1 cup Garlic Olive Tapenade (page 173)

1 cup thinly sliced yellow onion

1 whole lemon, seeded and thinly sliced

¼ cup Homemade Vegetable Bone Broth (page 162)

1 tablespoon capers

¼ teaspoon sea salt

½ teaspoon minced garlic

½ teaspoon chopped fresh oregano

1 teaspoon chopped fresh parsley

1 tablespoon extra-virgin olive oil

ONE-PAN

Prep time: 30 minutes
Cook time: 1 hour

Serving Tip: Serve over Garlic Mashed Rutabagas (page 69) for a traditional comfort food–style dinner.

1. Preheat the oven to 350°F.

2. Place the pork tenderloin on a cutting board. Using a sharp knife, make a horizontal cut ¼ inch from the bottom of the tenderloin, cutting through to within ¼ inch of the opposite edge. Unroll the tenderloin, exposing the cut surface. Continue cutting and unrolling to make a flat piece of meat.

3. Spread the pork flat on the cutting board. Cover the pork with a large piece of plastic wrap.

4. With the flat side of a meat mallet, gently pound the pork into a uniform thickness. Avoid excessive pounding, which will cause unwanted thin spots. Remove the plastic wrap.

5. Spread the tapenade evenly across the flat piece of pork, leaving an empty 1-inch strip across the top.

6. Starting with the closest edge to you, roll the pork toward the 1-inch strip of bare meat, trying to keep your roll as tight and uniform as possible. Set aside.

7. Place the sliced onion and lemon in the bottom of a Dutch oven or roasting pan, and add the broth and capers.

8. Gently place the pork roulade on top of the onion and lemon, seam-side down.

9. Sprinkle the salt, garlic, oregano, and parsley over the roulade and drizzle with the olive oil.

10. Bake uncovered for 45 minutes, or until the roulade reaches an internal temperature of 140°F.

11. Remove the pot from the oven, cover, and let the meat rest for 5 to 10 minutes, or until it reaches a final internal temperature of 145°F.

12. Slice the roulade into ½-inch-thick slices. Place the onion and lemon on a platter, gently place the sliced pork on top, and pour the pan juices over top just before serving.

Per Serving (¼ prepared recipe): Calories: 323; Total Fat: 23g; Saturated Fat: 4g; Sodium: 1,151mg; Carbohydrates: 11g; Fiber: 5g; Protein: 23g

Cilantro Lime Pork Carnitas

These carnitas are a great way to enjoy a Mexican-style dish and flavor while still avoiding nightshades like tomatoes and peppers. Instead, you'll rely on fresh cilantro and lime and grapefruit juices for a bold flavor. Cilantro is a powerful medicinal herb, packed with phytochemicals that may help remove harmful heavy metals from the blood. **MAKES 4 SERVINGS**

1 pound pork butt, cut into 2-inch cubes

¼ cup fresh cilantro leaves, packed

½ cup thinly sliced white onion

1 tablespoon minced garlic

3 tablespoons freshly squeezed lime juice

3 tablespoons freshly squeezed grapefruit juice

1 teaspoon salt

¼ teaspoon dried oregano

ONE-POT

Prep time: 10 minutes
Cook time: 4 hours

1. In a slow cooker, combine the pork, cilantro, onion, garlic, citrus juices, salt, and oregano.

2. Cook on high for 4 hours.

3. Shred the meat with two forks before serving.

Per Serving (4 ounces): Calories: 226; Total Fat: 14g; Saturated Fat: 5g; Sodium: 653mg; Carbohydrates: 4g; Fiber: 1g; Protein: 20g

Substitution Tip: Try this recipe with 1 pound of boneless, skinless chicken thighs. If you do not have lime or grapefruit juice, you can substitute freshly squeezed orange juice.

Serving Tip: Serve these carnitas inside Grain-Free Tortillas (page 174) or over From-Scratch Cauliflower Rice (page 60) topped with Quick Pickled Red Onions (page 48) and Creamy Coconut Milk Yogurt (page 177).

Balsamic Roasted Ham with Golden Beets

You can get an uncured ham from your local butcher or farm and make the perfect Sunday supper. The ham gets paired with sweet and savory golden beets and pears, making this dish an ideal combination of flavor and comfort. Golden beets contain many vitamins and minerals that studies have shown protect overall health, including vitamin A, beta-carotene, lycopene, and zeaxanthin.

MAKES 8 SERVINGS

½ pound golden beets, peeled and thinly sliced

2 pounds uncured ham, bone in or boneless

½ pound pears, peeled, cored, and thickly sliced

½ cup balsamic vinegar

1 tablespoon coconut sugar

5-INGREDIENT

Prep time: 10 minutes
Cook time: 2 hours

Ingredient Tip: If you can't find golden beets at the store, you can use regular beets or another root vegetable like rutabagas, turnips, carrots, or parsnips.

1. Preheat the oven to 300°F.

2. Place the beets in a Dutch oven. Place the ham on top of the beets.

3. Surround the ham with the pears.

4. In a small bowl, whisk together the balsamic vinegar and coconut sugar. Pour this mixture over the ham.

5. Roast for 2 hours, or until the ham's internal temperature reaches 150°F.

Per Serving (⅛ prepared recipe): Calories: 164; Total Fat: 4g; Saturated Fat: 1g; Sodium: 314mg; Carbohydrates: 7g; Fiber: 2g; Protein: 27g

Churrasco Skirt Steak with Chimichurri

Lean beef is a high-protein, nutrient-rich source of many essential vitamins and minerals such as iron, zinc, and vitamin B₆. Topped with a fresh, zesty chimi-churri sauce, this steak is the perfect centerpiece for any meal, and it can easily be sliced to make fajitas or other Mexican-inspired dishes. **MAKES 4 SERVINGS**

1 pound flank steak
1 teaspoon salt
1 teaspoon extra-virgin
  olive oil

½ cup Chimichurri
  Sauce (page 167)

**5-INGREDIENT
30-MINUTE
ONE-POT**

Prep time: 5 minutes
Cook time: 10 minutes
Rest time: 10 minutes

Substitution Tip: This cooking method works for many different types of lean steak, such as flank steak, and the steak can be topped with a variety of sauces for unique flavor combinations.

1. Generously season the flank steak on both sides with salt, then rub it on both sides with the olive oil.

2. Set a cast-iron skillet over medium-high heat.

3. Once the skillet is hot, add the flank steak and sear for 2 to 3 minutes per side, depending on the thickness of the meat, until it reaches an internal temperature of 125°F. Remove the meat from the skillet and wrap it tightly in foil.

4. Let the steak rest for 10 minutes, or until it reaches your desired internal temperature: 145°F for medium-rare, 160°F for medium, and 170°F for well-done.

5. Thinly slice the steak against the grain and top it with the sauce just before serving.

Per Serving (4 ounces steak): Calories: 188; Total Fat: 8g; Saturated Fat: 3g; Sodium: 798mg; Carbohydrates: 2g; Fiber: 0g; Protein: 25g

Stuffed Cabbage Rolls

Cabbage rolls are a delicious, hearty meal that the whole family will enjoy. Traditionally used in dishes like coleslaw or sauerkraut, cabbage has large leaves that also make the perfect wrap for seasoned ground beef. Cabbage is low in calories but high in important nutrients like vitamins C and K, and it contains powerful antioxidants like polyphenols and sulfur compounds. **MAKES 4 SERVINGS**

Olive oil cooking spray
1 pound ground beef
2 cups riced cauliflower
½ cup minced onion

2 teaspoons
  minced garlic
1 teaspoon salt
1 head green cabbage

5-INGREDIENT

Prep time: 30 minutes
Cook time: 45 minutes

1. Preheat the oven to 350°F. Set a large pot of water on the stove to boil.

2. Lightly grease a glass baking dish with cooking spray and set it aside.

3. Prepare an ice bath by filling a large bowl with ice and water. Set aside.

4. In another large bowl, combine the ground beef, riced cauliflower, onion, garlic, and salt. Set aside.

5. Core the cabbage and place it in the boiling water. Boil for 5 minutes, then transfer the cabbage to the ice bath.

6. When the cabbage is cool enough to handle, begin to gently remove the outside leaves and set them in a strainer. They should be soft and pliable.

7. Add ¼ cup of the meat mixture to the center of a cooked cabbage leaf.

continued

Serving Tip: Serve the cabbage rolls topped with Bone Broth Brown Gravy (page 164).

Ingredient Tip: In this recipe, it doesn't matter if the cauliflower rice is cooked ahead of time or not. If you already have From-Scratch Cauliflower Rice (page 60) prepared, you can use that.

8. Fold in the sides, then roll it up from the bottom to form the cabbage roll. Set the roll inside the greased baking dish. Repeat this process until all of the meat mixture has been used (you should have approximately 12 rolls).

9. Cover the baking dish with aluminum foil and bake for 45 minutes or until the filling is cooked through.

Per Serving (3 rolls): Calories: 225; Total Fat: 8g; Saturated Fat: 3g; Sodium: 614mg; Carbohydrates: 15g; Fiber: 6g; Protein: 25g

Baked Carrot Meatloaf

Meatloaf is a classic, cozy staple in the American diet, but it can be tricky to make without using eggs for a binder or bread for a filler. Thankfully, shredded carrots and minced mushrooms provide the delicious traditional taste and texture of meatloaf without those ingredients that can trigger inflammation in the body during this time of healing. **MAKES 8 SERVINGS**

Olive oil cooking spray

2 tablespoons extra-virgin olive oil

1 cup minced yellow onion

1 tablespoon minced garlic

2½ cups shredded carrots

1½ cups minced mushrooms

2 pounds ground beef

2 tablespoons coconut liquid aminos

3 tablespoons cassava flour

1 teaspoon dried thyme

MAKE-AHEAD

Prep time: 30 minutes
Cook time: 1 hour

1. Preheat the oven to 350°F. Lightly grease a loaf pan with cooking spray and set it aside.

2. In a large skillet over medium heat, warm the olive oil.

3. When the oil is hot, add the onion and sweat it for 2 minutes, or until slightly tender.

4. Stir in the garlic and cook, stirring frequently, for 1 minute.

5. Add the shredded carrots and sweat, stirring frequently, for another 2 minutes.

6. Add the minced mushrooms and cook, stirring occasionally, for 2 minutes, or until soft. Remove the mixture from the heat and allow it to cool.

continued

Make-Ahead Tip: There are several ways to prep and store this dish ahead of time. Put the meatloaf together and refrigerate, uncooked, for up to 3 days before baking. Or, bake the entire meatloaf, let it cool, and slice and freeze individual portions for up to 2 months. When ready to enjoy, thaw it in the refrigerator overnight before reheating in a skillet.

Ingredient Tip: To save time and energy, mince the yellow onion and mushrooms in a food processor. You can also shred large carrots using a food processor if you have the right attachment, or simply purchase matchstick or shredded carrots from the grocery store.

7. In a large bowl, mix together the vegetable mixture, ground beef, coconut aminos, cassava flour, and dried thyme. Be careful not to overwork the meat, as this will result in a tougher consistency.

8. Transfer the mixture to the greased loaf pan. Bake for 1 hour, or until an internal temperature of 165°F has been reached.

   Serving Tip: Serve this dish topped with Bone Broth Brown Gravy (page 164).

Per Serving (4 ounces): Calories: 223; Total Fat: 12g; Saturated Fat: 4g; Sodium: 115mg; Carbohydrates: 7g; Fiber: 1g; Protein: 23g

Seared Filet Mignon with Horseradish Cream

Having dietary restrictions shouldn't mean that you can't enjoy an indulgent meal on occasion as a celebration or special treat. This dish is sure to impress everyone in your household, with restrictions or not, while providing important nutrients to help your body heal and recover. **MAKES 4 SERVINGS**

1 teaspoon extra-virgin olive oil

2 (8-ounce) filet mignon steaks, cut in half for a total of 4 (4-ounce) filets

½ cup Creamy Coconut Milk Yogurt (page 177)

1 tablespoon grated fresh horseradish

5-INGREDIENT
30-MINUTE

Prep time: 10 minutes
Cook time: 15 minutes

Substitution Tip: If you don't have filet mignon, you can use other tender steak cuts, such as strip steak.

Serving Tip: Pair this entrée with the Sautéed Lemon Garlic Kale (page 62). The vitamin C from the lemon and kale will help your body absorb the iron from the steak more easily.

1. Preheat the oven to 400°F.

2. Gently rub the olive oil all over the filets to keep them from sticking to the pan.

3. Place a cast-iron or other oven-safe skillet over medium-high heat for 3 to 4 minutes, or until very hot. Add the filets and sear for 2 minutes.

4. Flip the filets and sear for an additional 2 minutes.

5. Place the skillet in the preheated oven and cook until the filets reach your desired internal temperature: 145°F for medium-rare, 160°F for medium, and 170°F for well-done.

6. Meanwhile, in a small bowl, whisk together the coconut milk yogurt and horseradish.

7. Gently spoon the horseradish cream over the cooked filets; serve immediately.

Per Serving (4 ounces filet with ⅛ cup prepared sauce): Calories: 304; Total Fat: 18g; Saturated Fat: 9g; Sodium: 89mg; Carbohydrates: 1g; Fiber: 0g; Protein: 32g

Sunday Supper Pot Roast

Pot roast is a classic dish that can bring back memories of cozy family dinners. With a few swaps, this dish can become AIP friendly. We bet no one will even notice that the rutabagas are not actually potatoes! **MAKES 4 TO 8 SERVINGS**

½ pound celery, cut into 2-inch pieces

2 white onions, cut into ½-inch-thick slices

1 tablespoon minced garlic

1 pound carrots, peeled and cut into 3-inch pieces

1½ pounds rutabagas, peeled and cut into 3-inch chunks

1 bay leaf

1 teaspoon dried thyme

1 teaspoon dried rosemary

1 teaspoon salt

2 pounds chuck roast

1½ cups Homemade Vegetable Bone Broth (page 162)

MAKE-AHEAD

Prep time: 30 minutes
Cook time: 6 hours

Make-Ahead Tip: This easy meal will make more than 4 servings, helping you meal prep for the week ahead. Simply portion the uneaten meat and vegetables into individual airtight (preferably glass) containers and refrigerate for use throughout the week.

1. In a slow cooker, arrange the celery, onions, and garlic, followed by the carrots and rutabagas.

2. Add the bay leaf, thyme, and rosemary.

3. Sprinkle the salt on both sides of the roast.

4. Heat a large skillet over medium-high heat. Allow the pan to get very hot.

5. Add the roast to the hot pan and sear for 1 minute. Keep turning the roast to sear for 1 minute on each side.

6. Place the chuck roast in the slow cooker on top of the vegetables.

7. Cook on low for 6 hours, or until the meat is cooked through and easily falls apart with a fork.

Per Serving (4 ounces meat): Calories: 232; Total Fat: 7g; Saturated Fat: 2g; Sodium: 129mg; Carbohydrates: 16g; Fiber: 5g; Protein: 26g

Portobello Mushroom Beef Burgers

These mouthwatering burgers have been given an adult upgrade with the addition of mushrooms. Mushrooms contain nutrients important for managing Hashimoto's. Mushrooms are rich in selenium, a mineral that studies have connected to proper thyroid function. **MAKES 4 SERVINGS**

2 tablespoons
    extra-virgin olive oil
½ cup minced
    yellow onion
1 tablespoon
    minced garlic

2 cups puréed white
    mushrooms
2 pounds ground beef
½ teaspoon salt

5-INGREDIENT
30-MINUTE
MAKE-AHEAD

Prep time: 10 minutes
Cook time: 20 minutes

1. Heat the olive oil in a large skillet over medium heat.

2. Add the onion and sauté for 2 to 3 minutes, or until golden brown.

3. Add the garlic and cook, stirring frequently, for 1 minute.

4. Add the mushrooms and cook, stirring frequently, until most of the moisture is gone, approximately 10 minutes. Turn off the heat and allow the mixture to cool.

5. Once the mushroom mixture has cooled, scrape it into a large bowl, add the ground beef and salt, and mix well.

6. Form the mixture into 4 large or 8 small patties (see Cooking Tip).

7. Return the patties to the skillet over medium heat and cook for 2 to 3 minutes per side, or to your desired doneness. (For a well-done burger, aim for an internal temperature of 165°F.)

Make-Ahead Tip: You can make the burger mix and form the patties in advance. Wrap the patties individually in wax paper and store them in the refrigerator for up to 5 days. For longer storage, place the individually wrapped patties in an airtight container and freeze them for up to 2 months.

Cooking Tip: You can make sliders or traditional-size burgers, depending on your preference. To make sliders, form 8 (2-ounce) patties; to make regular burgers, form 4 (4-ounce) patties.

Per Serving (4 ounces): Calories: 396; Total Fat: 23g; Saturated Fat: 7g; Sodium: 464mg; Carbohydrates: 3g; Fiber: 1g; Protein: 45g

Mediterranean Lamb Meatballs

Lamb is a staple lean protein in any Mediterranean-style diet, particularly in Greek cuisine. On average, a 3-ounce serving of lamb has only 150 calories. Naturally protein-packed, this nutrient-rich red meat is composed of nearly 40 percent heart-healthy monounsaturated fatty acids, making it an excellent meat option. **MAKES 8 SERVINGS**

2 pounds ground lamb

½ cup minced red onion

½ cup minced kalamata olives

¼ cup chopped fresh parsley

1 teaspoon chopped fresh mint

1 teaspoon chopped fresh oregano

½ teaspoon salt

2 tablespoons coconut oil or avocado oil

30-MINUTE
MAKE-AHEAD

Prep time: 20 minutes
Cook time: 10 minutes

Make-Ahead Tip: The meatballs can be prepared through step 2 and frozen. When ready to use, thaw them in the refrigerator for one day before picking up the recipe at step 3.

Ingredient Tip: You can substitute ground beef for the ground lamb in this recipe.

1. In a large bowl, combine the lamb, onion, olives, parsley, mint, oregano, and salt, using your hands to mix everything together.

2. Once the meat mixture is well combined, roll it into 1-inch meatballs. Set aside.

3. Heat the olive oil in a large cast-iron skillet over medium heat. Carefully arrange the meatballs in the skillet so they are not touching each other. Work in batches if needed.

4. Increase the heat to medium-high. (If necessary, use a splatter screen to protect yourself from the hot oil.)

5. Cook the meatballs for 3 to 4 minutes on the first side, or until they easily release from the bottom of the pan.

6. Flip the meatballs and cook on the other side for 3 to 4 minutes, rotating as necessary to ensure an even crust, until they reach an internal temperature of 155°F.

Per Serving (3 meatballs): Calories: 363; Total Fat: 31g; Saturated Fat: 15g; Sodium: 287mg; Carbohydrates: 2g; Fiber: 1g; Protein: 20g

Lamb Kebabs with Mint Yogurt Sauce

A single portion of lamb provides more than half of your daily protein needs, making it an ideal fuel for healing bodies. With a variety of essential vitamins and minerals, including iron, vitamin B_{12}, niacin, zinc, selenium, riboflavin, and even alpha-linolenic acid, an important omega-3 fatty acid, lamb is clearly a nutrient-dense choice. **MAKES 4 SERVINGS**

1 pound boneless leg of lamb, cut into 1-inch cubes

8 (10-inch) metal skewers (or wooden skewers soaked in water for 30 minutes)

2 cups peeled, cored, and diced Granny Smith apples

1 cup pearl onions

1 teaspoon salt

1 tablespoon extra-virgin olive oil, plus more for the grill

½ cup Creamy Ranch Dressing (page 172)

½ cup fresh mint leaves, packed

5-INGREDIENT
30-MINUTE

Prep time: 10 minutes
Cook time: 10 minutes
Rest time: 10 minutes

Cooking Tip: No grill? No problem. Simply cook the skewers on a hot cast-iron pan over high heat, following steps 4 and 5.

1. Thread the cubes of lamb onto the skewers, alternating with the diced apples and pearl onions.

2. Apply a liberal amount of salt to both sides of the lamb skewers and brush them with the olive oil.

3. Prepare an outdoor grill for high heat and liberally oil the grill grate with more olive oil.

4. Carefully lay the skewers on the oiled grill grate. Grill for 2 to 3 minutes, flip the skewers, and then grill for another 2 to 4 minutes, or until the lamb reaches an internal temperature of 155°F.

5. Remove the skewers from the grill and wrap them tightly in foil. Let the meat rest for approximately 10 minutes, or until it reaches an internal temperature of 165°F.

6. While the meat is resting, in a small food processor, blend together the ranch dressing and fresh mint.

7. Top the skewers with the sauce just before serving.

Per Serving (2 skewers): Calories: 412; Total Fat: 29g; Saturated Fat: 20g; Sodium: 364mg; Carbohydrates: 19g; Fiber: 4g; Protein: 21g

Lamb and Vegetable Stew

This wonderful stew brings together all the nutritious benefits of vegetables, lean protein, and broth for a comforting, nourishing bowl of goodness that is delicious anytime of day. Bone broth is especially beneficial because it is made with animal bones; it gets its healing properties from the collagen and nutrients that are extracted during the long cooking process. Studies have shown that collagen, the most abundant protein in the body, may help with many issues, from alleviating joint pain to improving skin ailments. **MAKES 4 SERVINGS**

2 tablespoons extra-virgin olive oil, divided

1 pound lamb stew meat, cut into 1-inch chunks

1 teaspoon salt, divided

2 cups peeled and diced sweet potatoes

1 cup diced white onion

1 cup peeled and diced carrots

1 cup diced celery

1 tablespoon minced garlic

6 cups Homemade Vegetable Bone Broth (page 162)

2 bay leaves

2 cups chopped kale leaves

1 tablespoon chopped fresh parsley

ONE-POT

Prep time: 20 minutes
Cook time: 1 hour

Substitution Tip: Feel free to use a variety of vegetables or dark leafy greens, depending on what you have on hand.

1. Heat 1 tablespoon of olive oil in a large soup pot over medium heat.

2. Season the meat with ½ teaspoon of salt. Add the meat to the pot and cook until browned, 4 to 5 minutes. Transfer the meat to a plate and set it aside.

3. Add the remaining 1 tablespoon of olive oil, the sweet potatoes, onion, carrots, celery, and garlic. Sauté for 5 minutes, stirring frequently.

4. Return the meat to the pot along with the broth, bay leaves, and remaining ½ teaspoon of salt. Bring the broth to a boil, then reduce the heat and simmer for 45 minutes, or until the meat is very tender.

5. Add the chopped kale and simmer for an additional 2 minutes, just until wilted.

6. Remove the bay leaves and garnish with the parsley just before serving.

Per Serving (1 cup): Calories: 343; Total Fat: 13g; Saturated Fat: 3g; Sodium: 605mg; Carbohydrates: 31g; Fiber: 4g; Protein: 25g

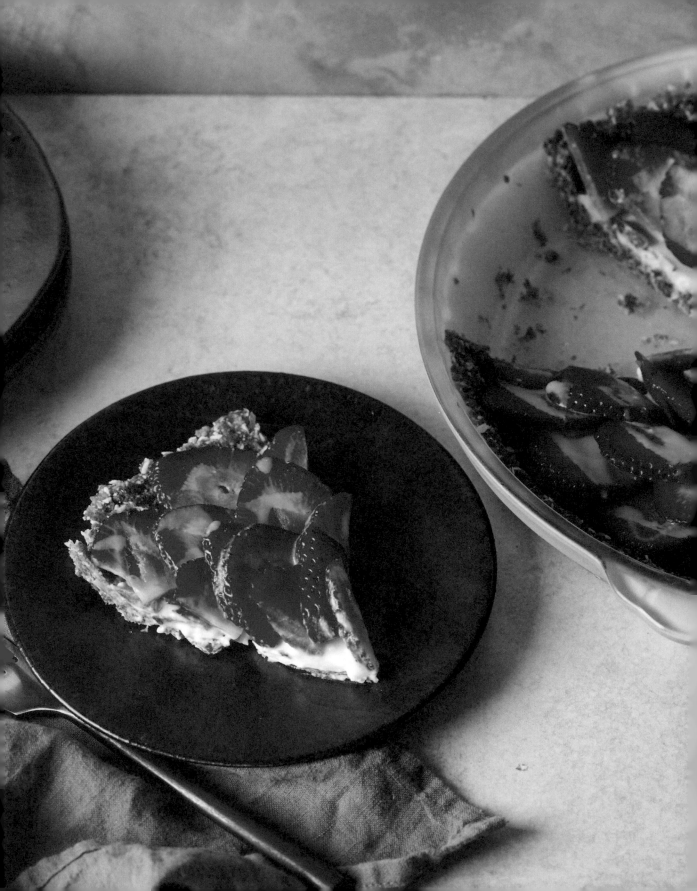

8 *Snacks and Sweet Treats*

Apricot Date Energy Bites

Dates, the fruit of the date palm tree, have a chewy texture and sweet flavor. High in dietary fiber, dates also contain phosphorus, potassium, calcium, and magnesium. Because dates are dried, they are more concentrated in calories and in sweetness—in fact, they serve as a popular all-natural sweetener. This means you don't need to add any additional sugar or sweetener and should enjoy these bites in moderation. **MAKES 12 ENERGY BITES**

¾ cup pitted dates

¾ cup unsweetened dried apricots

¾ cup unsweetened dried cranberries

2 tablespoons unflavored collagen peptides

1 tablespoon coconut oil

5-INGREDIENT
30-MINUTE
ONE-BOWL

Prep time: 10 minutes

1. Combine the dates, apricots, and cranberries in a food processor and process on high for 30 to 60 seconds, or until the fruit is broken down and a "dough" starts to form.

2. Add the collagen peptides and coconut oil; pulse for another 30 seconds.

3. Remove the mixture from the food processor and shape it into 1-inch balls.

4. Enjoy immediately or store the balls in an airtight container in the refrigerator for up to 7 days.

Ingredient Tip: Try different unsweetened dried fruits for varying flavor combinations. Options include dried figs, dried blueberries, dried cherries, and more.

Per Serving (2 bites): Calories: 124; Total Fat: 2g; Saturated Fat: 2g; Sodium: 0mg; Carbohydrates: 24g; Fiber: 2g; Protein: 4g

Caramel Date Sauce

When cooked down, dates melt to create a deliciously sweet, caramel-like sauce. Dates are a good source of energy, naturally occurring sugars, and dietary fiber. These delicious fruits also provide many essential minerals, such as calcium, iron, phosphorus, and zinc, which some studies suggest can help strengthen bone health. **MAKES 4 SERVINGS**

1 (14-ounce) can full-fat coconut milk

¾ cup pitted dates, diced

4 apples, peeled, cored, and sliced

5-INGREDIENT
30-MINUTE
MAKE-AHEAD
ONE-POT

Prep time: 10 minutes
Cook time: 30 minutes

1. In a small saucepan over medium-high heat, combine the coconut milk and dates. Bring the liquid to a boil and let it boil for 30 seconds, stirring constantly.

2. Reduce the heat to low and simmer uncovered, stirring occasionally, for 30 minutes, or until the sauce has thickened (see Cooking Tip).

3. Remove the pan from the heat and serve the sauce with the apple slices for dipping.

Per Serving (2 tablespoons, 1 apple): Calories: 401; Total Fat: 24g; Saturated Fat: 21g; Sodium: 16mg; Carbohydrates: 52g; Fiber: 10g; Protein: 3g

Make-Ahead Tip: Prepare the sauce ahead of time and store it in a sealed container in the refrigerator for up to 14 days. Warm it slightly before serving, if desired.

Cooking Tip: You can cook the sauce to the consistency of your choice. Keep it thinner for a free-flowing sauce, or cook it longer for a thick, almost nut-butter-like consistency.

Cinnamon Tapioca Pudding

You might have fond memories of tapioca pudding from your childhood, but you may have never known that tapioca is actually derived from the cassava tuber, which appears often in this book in its flour form. Cassava flour is naturally allergen-friendly, making it an ideal option for those following the autoimmune protocol. Although desserts and sweet treats should be enjoyed in moderation to minimize blood sugar spikes, it's nice to have a sweet and comforting dessert option on hand. **MAKES 4 SERVINGS**

3 tablespoons quick-cooking tapioca

⅓ cup coconut sugar

2 tablespoons unflavored collagen peptides

1 teaspoon ground cinnamon

2 (14-ounce) cans light coconut milk

1 teaspoon pure vanilla extract

⅛ teaspoon salt

30-MINUTE
ONE-POT

Prep time: 5 minutes
Cook time: 25 minutes

Ingredient Tip: This recipe is made with quick-cooking tapioca, which is already broken down. The consistency will be smoother than a traditional tapioca pudding.

1. In a medium saucepan, combine the tapioca, coconut sugar, collagen peptides, cinnamon, and coconut milk. Stir well and let stand for 5 minutes.

2. Place the pan over medium heat. Bring the mixture to a boil, stirring constantly. Boil for 1 minute, then turn off the heat and stir in the vanilla and salt.

3. Allow to stand for 20 minutes before serving warm or chilled.

Per Serving (½ cup): Calories: 254; Total Fat: 10g; Saturated Fat: 9g; Sodium: 638mg; Carbohydrates: 40g; Fiber: 0g; Protein: 5g

Creamy Banana Pudding

One of the most popular fruits on the planet, bananas contain many nutrients, including potassium, magnesium, folate, and vitamin A. They are also rich in fiber and important minerals that help regulate blood pressure, so a moderate amount of the fruit is an excellent addition to any diet. **MAKES 4 SERVINGS**

1 (14-ounce) can light coconut milk

2 ripe bananas

1 teaspoon pure vanilla extract

1 tablespoon unflavored beef gelatin

½ (11.25-ounce) can sweetened condensed coconut milk

5-INGREDIENT
30-MINUTE

Prep time: 10 minutes
Cook time: 20 minutes

Serving Tip: Serve this pudding inside the date crust from the Strawberry Fruit Tart (page 152) for an upgraded banana cream pie.

1. In a food processor, combine the light coconut milk, bananas, and vanilla. Process on high for 30 seconds, or until smooth. Transfer to a large saucepan.

2. Sprinkle the gelatin over the milk and banana mixture and allow it to "bloom" for 5 minutes.

3. Place the saucepan over medium-high heat and bring the liquid to a boil. Cook, stirring constantly, for 30 seconds, then reduce the heat to low.

4. Stir in the sweetened condensed coconut milk, increase the heat to medium-low, and cook for 5 minutes, being careful not to let the mixture boil.

5. Remove the pan from the heat and pour the pudding into individual containers or one large container. Refrigerate for at least 2 hours before serving.

Per Serving (½ cup): Calories: 248; Total Fat: 9g; Saturated Fat: 9g; Sodium: 54mg; Carbohydrates: 40g; Fiber: 2g; Protein: 3g

Two-Ingredient Grape Gelatin

Collagen is a natural protein; in fact, it's the most abundant protein in the body. It's also an important nutrient to consume when healing the gut because it is beneficial to overall gut health. Additionally, studies have shown that collagen may help maintain healthy joints, support bone strength, and support the health and vitality of skin, hair, and nails. Gelatin provides collagen in the form of amino acids. When paired with a high-quality, 100 percent pure fruit juice that can provide antioxidants, this dessert suddenly becomes as nutritious as it is delicious. **MAKES 4 SERVINGS**

4 cups 100% pure Concord grape juice (no sugar added), divided

2½ tablespoons unflavored beef gelatin

5-INGREDIENT

Cook time: 10 minutes
Rest time: 3 hours

1. Pour 2 cups of grape juice into a medium bowl. Sprinkle the gelatin over the juice. Set the bowl aside to allow the gelatin to bloom.

2. Pour the remaining 2 cups of grape juice into a small saucepan over medium heat. Use a digital instant-read thermometer to bring the juice to 200°F, or just before boiling. Do not allow the juice to boil.

3. Carefully pour the hot juice into the bowl with the juice and gelatin mixture. Stir well to dissolve the gelatin.

4. Pour the gelatin mixture into a glass bowl, dish, or mold. Refrigerate for 3 to 6 hours, or until firm.

5. Cut into cubes and serve.

Ingredient Tip: You can use any 100% pure juice option you like in this recipe, but try to aim for one with the most nutrition and antioxidants available, like blueberry juice, pomegranate juice, or tart cherry juice.

Per Serving (¼ prepared recipe): Calories: 155; Total Fat: 0g; Saturated Fat: 0g; Sodium: 39mg; Carbohydrates: 34g; Fiber: 0g; Protein: 4g

Honey Cinnamon Fruit Salad

Also called a drupe, a stone fruit has a stone, or pit, inside. Peaches, nectarines, plums, lychees, mangos, and cherries all fit into this category, and they all offer a range of beneficial nutrients including dietary fiber and antioxidants. They're enhanced in this recipe with some added sweetness and flavor. **MAKES 4 SERVINGS**

4 cups pitted and diced stone fruit of choice

2 tablespoons raw honey

½ teaspoon pure vanilla extract

¼ teaspoon ground cinnamon

⅛ teaspoon salt

5-INGREDIENT
30-MINUTE
ONE-BOWL

Prep time: 10 minutes
Rest time: 5 minutes

1. In a large bowl, gently toss together the fruit, honey, vanilla, cinnamon, and salt.

2. Let rest for 5 minutes to marry the flavors before serving.

Per Serving (1 cup): Calories: 93; Total Fat: 0g; Saturated Fat: 0g; Sodium: 35mg; Carbohydrates: 23g; Fiber: 2g; Protein: 1g

Recipe Tip: To add depth of flavor, use a mix of stone fruits, such as peaches, plums, and cherries.

Tropical Mango Gelato

Gone are the days of delicious frozen treats made only from dairy products. This sorbet is made by blending mango and coconuts, two tropical fruits that create an ultra-smooth, creamy texture when frozen and blended. Like dates and olives, mangos and coconuts are members of the drupe family. They're rich in antioxidants such as zeaxanthin and have anti-inflammatory properties.

MAKES 4 SERVINGS

2 cups frozen
   mango chunks
1 (14-ounce) can
   coconut milk
¼ cup pure maple syrup
½ teaspoon pure
   vanilla extract
⅛ teaspoon ground
   turmeric

**5-INGREDIENT
30-MINUTE**

Prep time: 10 minutes
Freezing time: 10 minutes

1. In a high-speed blender or food processor, combine the frozen mango, coconut milk, maple syrup, vanilla, and turmeric.
2. Blend on high speed for 3 minutes, stopping to scrape down the sides as needed.
3. Place the sorbet in a freezer-safe container and freeze for 10 minutes before serving.

Substitution Tip: Try this recipe with frozen pineapple instead of frozen mango for a new take on Disney's classic treat, the Dole Whip.

Per Serving (½ cup): Calories: 333; Total Fat: 24g; Saturated Fat: 21g; Sodium: 18mg; Carbohydrates: 32g; Fiber: 4g; Protein: 3g

Coconut Fried Apples

As the old saying goes, "An apple a day keeps the doctor away." Apples are, in fact, a very healthy fruit that provide antioxidants, phytonutrients, dietary fiber, and beneficial prebiotics to nourish the good bacteria in the digestive tract. They are also delicious when caramelized naturally by heat. **MAKES 4 SERVINGS**

2 tablespoons
   coconut oil
4 cups sliced apples

2 tablespoons
   coconut sugar
1 tablespoon
   filtered water

5-INGREDIENT
30-MINUTE
ONE-POT

Prep time: 5 minutes
Cook time: 10 minutes

1. In a medium skillet over medium heat, melt the coconut oil.

2. Carefully add the sliced apples and cook for 5 to 7 minutes, stirring frequently, until they are nicely caramelized.

3. Stir in the coconut sugar and filtered water. Cook for 1 minute, then remove the skillet from the heat.

Per Serving (¼ prepared recipe): Calories: 197; Total Fat: 7g; Saturated Fat: 6g; Sodium: 2mg; Carbohydrates: 37g; Fiber: 5g; Protein: 1g

Ingredient Tip: You can use any type of apple in this dish, but be sure to use apples that work best for cooking so they stay firm and don't get mushy. Consider varieties like Granny Smith, Fuji, Honeycrisp, or Braeburn.

Slow Cooker Poached Pears

Fruit makes the perfect dessert on the AIP because it helps satisfy a sweet tooth while also providing nutrients that facilitate healing. Pears deliver vitamin C, vitamin K, potassium, calcium, iron, magnesium, and folate. Plus, if the skin is left on, it can provide nearly 6 grams, or 24 percent, of your recommended daily value for dietary fiber. **MAKES 4 SERVINGS**

1 cup filtered water
4 large pears, halved
  and cored

2 cinnamon sticks
2 tablespoons
  coconut sugar

**5-INGREDIENT
ONE-POT**

Prep time: 5 minutes
Cook time: 45 minutes

1. Pour the water into a slow cooker.
2. Add the pears and cinnamon sticks. Sprinkle with the coconut sugar.
3. Cover and cook on high for 45 minutes, or until the pears are tender.
4. Remove the cinnamon sticks before serving.

Per Serving (1 pear): Calories: 143; Total Fat: 0g; Saturated Fat: 0g; Sodium: 3mg; Carbohydrates: 38g; Fiber: 7g; Protein: 1g

Recipe Tip: Although some people don't like the texture of cooked pear skins, others enjoy it, or at least they choose to keep the skin on for the added dietary fiber and nutrients. Peel or don't peel based on your personal preference.

Ingredient Tip: This recipe can also be made with apples.

Raspberry Peach Fruit Leather

Fruit leather is a nutrient-dense snack for enjoying on-the-go, making it a perfect candidate for meal prep. Because it is a concentrated source of energy in the form of calories and sugar, you should enjoy this treat in moderation.

MAKES 4 SERVINGS

2 cups peeled and
 sliced peaches
2 cups fresh raspberries

2 tablespoons
 coconut sugar
2 tablespoons freshly
 squeezed lemon juice

1. Preheat the oven to 170°F.
2. Cover a baking sheet with a large piece of parchment paper (big enough to overlap the edges of the pan). Set aside.
3. In a food processor, purée the peaches, raspberries, sugar, and lemon juice until smooth.
4. Optional step: If you do not want seeds in your fruit leather, run the purée through a fine-mesh sieve to remove the seeds.
5. Pour the mixture onto the lined baking sheet. Place on the top rack of the oven, leaving the door slightly ajar. Cook for 5 hours.
6. The fruit leather is ready when the fruit is dry on the surface and no longer tacky. You should be able to easily cut it into strips.

Per Serving (¼ prepared recipe): Calories: 60; Total Fat: 1g; Saturated Fat: 0g; Sodium: 6mg; Carbohydrates: 14g; Fiber: 4g; Protein: 1g

**5-INGREDIENT
MAKE-AHEAD**

Prep time: 10 minutes
Cook time: 5 hours

Make-Ahead Tip: To store, make rollups: Roll the fruit leather in plastic wrap or parchment paper and store it in an airtight container at room temperature.

Ingredient Tip: Fruit leather can be made from any puréed fruit, so get creative! Try blueberry lemon or apple cinnamon depending on what's in season.

Strawberry Fruit Tart

Just because you're following the AIP doesn't mean you shouldn't have a delicious dessert recipe to enjoy and wow your friends and family with. This tart will do just that, while also providing helpful nutrients. If possible, use seasonal fruits to maximize freshness and nutrient density. **MAKES 4 SERVINGS**

1 teaspoon coconut oil, plus more for greasing

1 cup pitted dates

½ cup unsweetened coconut flakes

1 tablespoon coconut flour

¼ cup coconut cream

1 cup fresh strawberries, hulled and sliced

1 tablespoon sweetened condensed coconut milk

1 teaspoon boiling water

30-MINUTE

Prep time: 20 minutes
Rest time: 10 minutes

Ingredient Tip: Use any combination of berries and fruits to make this tart more versatile. Raspberries, blueberries, blackberries, and peaches all make excellent options.

1. Grease a pie dish with coconut oil and set it aside.

2. In a food processor, combine the dates, coconut flakes, coconut flour, and 1 teaspoon of coconut oil. Purée for 30 to 60 seconds, or until a "dough" begins to form.

3. Transfer the mixture to the greased pie dish. Using your hands, press the dough into a flat, even crust.

4. Spread the coconut cream evenly over the crust. Top with the sliced berries.

5. In a small bowl, whisk together the condensed coconut milk and boiling water. Pour this mixture evenly over the sliced berries.

6. Refrigerate for 10 minutes before serving.

Per Serving (¼ prepared recipe): Calories: 301; Total Fat: 15g; Saturated Fat: 12g; Sodium: 3mg; Carbohydrates: 44g; Fiber: 7g; Protein: 3g

Cherry Tigernut Flour Cookies

Tigernuts, which are actually not nuts at all, are small root vegetables native to Northern Africa and the Mediterranean. They are nut-free, as well as gluten- and grain-free, making them a perfect option for the AIP. Tigernuts contain dietary fiber, protein, iron, magnesium, zinc, and vitamin E. You should be able to find tigernut flour in your local grocery or health food store, thanks to its increasing popularity.

MAKES 8 COOKIES

1 cup tigernut flour

¼ cup tapioca flour

2 tablespoons unflavored collagen peptides

⅛ teaspoon baking soda

⅛ teaspoon salt

¼ cup full-fat coconut milk

2 tablespoons coconut oil, melted

2 tablespoons pure maple syrup

3 tablespoons unsweetened dried cherries

30-MINUTE

Prep time: 10 minutes
Cook time: 15 minutes

Variation Tip: You can omit the dried cherries altogether or use different types of dried fruit for more cookie variations.

1. Preheat the oven to 350°F. Line a baking sheet with aluminum foil and set it aside.

2. In a large bowl, whisk together the tigernut flour, tapioca flour, collagen peptides, baking soda, and salt. Set aside.

continued

3. In a small bowl, whisk together the coconut milk, coconut oil, and maple syrup.

4. Pour the wet ingredients into the dry and stir until well combined. Gently fold in the dried cherries.

5. Scoop tablespoon-size portions of dough onto the prepared baking sheet, spacing them evenly.

6. Bake for 12 to 15 minutes, or until the cookies are golden brown.

Per Serving (2 cookies): Calories: 135; Total Fat: 8g; Saturated Fat: 5g; Sodium: 455mg; Carbohydrates: 13g; Fiber: 3g; Protein: 2g

Baked Coconut Macaroon Bites

The health-promoting qualities of coconuts and coconut-based products have been debated. Though coconuts are high in saturated fat, these drupe fruits contain a unique combination of fatty acids known as medium-chain triglycerides, which many scientists believe to be beneficial to health. About 50 percent of the fatty acids in coconut oil are lauric acid, which has been found to kill harmful microorganisms in the body. **MAKES 12 COOKIES**

1½ cups unsweetened coconut flakes

¼ cup full-fat coconut milk

¼ cup sweetened condensed coconut milk (see Ingredient Tip)

5-INGREDIENT
30-MINUTE

Prep time: 10 minutes
Cook time: 10 minutes

1. Preheat the oven to 325°F. Line a baking sheet with aluminum foil and set it aside.

2. In a large bowl, mix together the coconut flakes, coconut milk, and condensed coconut milk.

3. Shape the dough into 1-inch balls and place them on the prepared baking sheet, spaced evenly.

4. Gently press down on the balls with your fingers or a fork to create ½-inch-thick cookies.

5. Bake for 15 minutes, or until slightly golden brown.

6. Allow the cookies to cool completely before serving.

Ingredient Tip: If you don't have sweetened condensed coconut milk, mix 2 tablespoons of coconut sugar with enough full-fat coconut milk to make ¼ cup.

Per Serving (2 cookies): Calories: 238; Total Fat: 19g; Saturated Fat: 16g; Sodium: 11mg; Carbohydrates: 13g; Fiber: 4g; Protein: 2g

Homemade Cherry Gummies

Gummy bears, that classic childhood candy favorite, just got an adult makeover with the use of unflavored beef gelatin. Unlike the gelatin you may typically purchase at the store, grass-fed bovine gelatin powder contains many important amino acids that may help support gut health. With the addition of honey and tart cherry juice, which has been shown to fight inflammation, these gummies are anything but average. **MAKES 4 SERVINGS**

1 cup unsweetened tart
   cherry juice

8 teaspoons unflavored
   beef gelatin powder
1 tablespoon raw honey

5-INGREDIENT

Prep time: 10 minutes
Cook time: 15 minutes
Freeze time: 15 minutes

1. Pour the cherry juice into a small saucepan and sprinkle with the gelatin. Allow to stand and thicken for 2 minutes.

2. Stir the mixture and turn the heat to medium-low. Cook, constantly stirring, until the liquid reaches a temperature of 165°F, about 5 minutes. Stir in the honey.

3. Carefully pour the hot liquid into your mold of choice.

4. Place the filled mold in the freezer for 15 minutes.

5. Remove from the freezer, cut into shapes if desired, and enjoy.

Per Serving (¼ prepared recipe): Calories: 59; Total Fat: 0g; Saturated Fat: 0g; Sodium: 18mg; Carbohydrates: 10g; Fiber: 0g; Protein: 5g

Serving Tip: Although having a dedicated gummy bear mold may be cute and helpful, it's not necessary. You can make this recipe in just about any container that you have; cut it to the desired shape and size once the mixture is set.

Substitution Tip: You can substitute any juice for the tart cherry juice in this recipe to achieve various flavor combinations. Just be sure to use 100 percent pure juice with no added sugar or other ingredients.

Homemade Coconut Whipped Cream with Fresh Berries

This recipe takes a little bit of advance planning, because you need to refrigerate the coconut milk overnight and freeze the bowl and beaters ahead of time. Once those steps are completed, though, you are less than 10 minutes away from coconut whipped cream that can be enjoyed with fresh berries or your favorite AIC-friendly dessert. **MAKES 4 SERVINGS**

1 (14-ounce) can full-fat coconut milk, refrigerated overnight

1 teaspoon coconut sugar

½ teaspoon pure vanilla extract

2 cups hulled and sliced strawberries

5-INGREDIENT

Prep time: 24 hours
Cook time: 5 minutes

Cooking Tip: Feel free to experiment with flavorings other than vanilla. For example, try mint extract, almond extract, lemon zest, matcha powder, or ground cinnamon.

1. Place a metal mixing bowl and the metal beaters from a hand mixer in the freezer at least 1 hour before you plan to make the whipped cream.

2. Open the can of coconut milk and scoop the cream solids into the cold mixing bowl. Be careful not to mix the solids with the liquid. Discard or reserve the remaining coconut milk liquid for another use.

3. Remove the beaters from the freezer and beat the coconut cream on medium speed for 1 minute. Turn to high speed and beat for 7 to 8 minutes, or until stiff peaks form.

4. Add the coconut sugar and vanilla extract and beat for 1 minute.

5. Serve immediately with the strawberries.

Per Serving (2 tablespoons): Calories: 136; Total Fat: 10g; Saturated Fat: 8g; Sodium: 1mg; Carbohydrates: 11g; Fiber: 2g; Protein: 2g

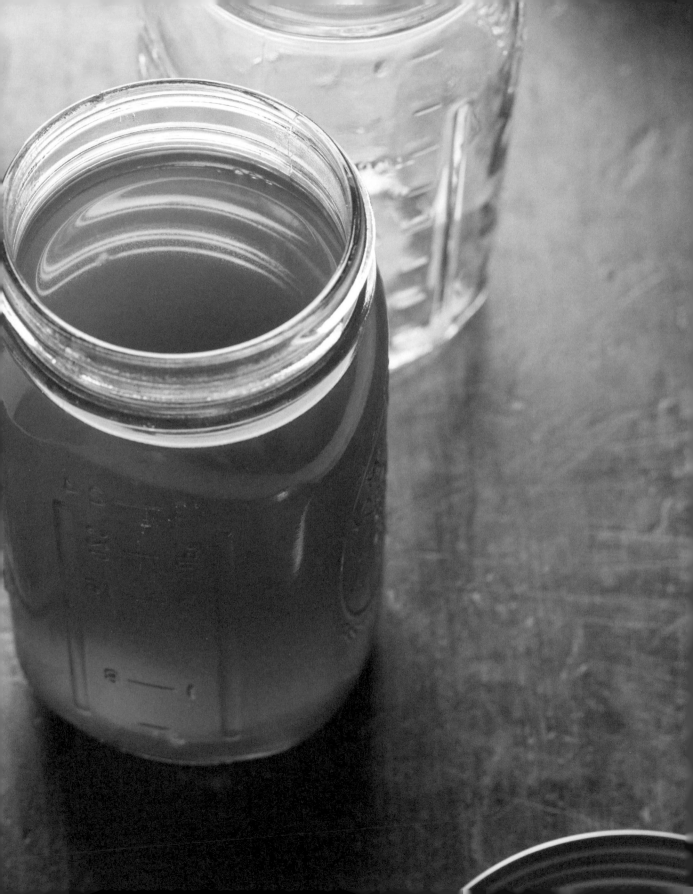

9 Sauces, Dressings, and Staples

AIP Spice Blend

Seasoning your food can be tricky on the AIP, because quite a few spices are off limits. Thankfully, this spice blend provides plenty of flavor that can be enjoyed on just about any savory dish, from roasted vegetables to meats and more.

MAKES ¼ CUP

1 tablespoon
   kosher salt

1 tablespoon dried
   rosemary

1 tablespoon
   dried parsley

2 teaspoons
   garlic powder

1½ teaspoons
   dried sage

½ teaspoon
   onion powder

5-INGREDIENT
30-MINUTE
MAKE-AHEAD
ONE-BOWL

Prep time: 10 minutes

Make-Ahead Tip: You can easily double or quadruple this recipe to store in the pantry for future use.

Serving Tip: Enjoy this spice blend in a variety of dishes, including Herbed Whole Roasted Cauliflower (page 65).

1. Using a mortar and pestle or a spice grinder, grind together the salt, rosemary, parsley, garlic powder, sage, and onion powder until the mixture resembles a fine powder.

2. Store at room temperature in a Mason jar with a tight-fitting lid for up to 2 months.

Per Serving (2 teaspoons): Calories: 6; Total Fat: 0g; Saturated Fat: 0g; Sodium: 241mg; Carbohydrates: 1g; Fiber: 0g; Protein: 0g

AIP-Friendly Ketchup

Ketchup without nightshades? It may seem impossible, but thankfully there are plenty of other delicious fruits and vegetables that can come together to make this perfect AIP-Friendly Ketchup. Elevated with the sweetness of beets and the tartness of plums, this recipe provides that classic ketchup taste you may be missing. **MAKES 2 CUPS**

2 cups sliced carrots

1½ cups diced
   unripe plums

½ cup diced beets

½ cup diced white onion

2 garlic cloves

1 tablespoon apple
   cider vinegar

2 teaspoons brown
   coconut sugar

1 teaspoon salt

1 tablespoon
   filtered water

MAKE-AHEAD

Prep time: 10 minutes
Cook time: 6 hours

1. In a small slow cooker, combine the carrots, plums, beets, onion, garlic, vinegar, coconut sugar, and salt.

2. Cook on high for 6 hours.

3. Transfer the contents to a food processor.

4. Blend until smooth, adding the water while blending, until the desired consistency is achieved.

Per Serving (1 tablespoon): Calories: 11; Total Fat: 0g; Saturated Fat: 0g; Sodium: 81mg; Carbohydrates: 3g; Fiber: 0g; Protein: 0g

Ingredient Tip: Unripe plums will add the sour and tangy flavor needed to mimic that of the tomatoes in traditional ketchup. Ripe plums will be sweeter and add a sweeter flavor.

Serving Tip: Add 1 teaspoon grated fresh horseradish and 1 teaspoon freshly squeezed lemon juice to 1 cup of this ketchup to make an AIP-friendly cocktail sauce.

Make-Ahead Tip: This ketchup can be stored in a Mason jar with a tight-fitting lid in the refrigerator for up to 7 days. If you're worried you won't use it all in a week, freeze some in ice cube trays so you can remove as much as you need in the future without waste.

Homemade Vegetable Bone Broth

Bone broth is touted for its amazing health benefits and has been a staple of most food cultures for centuries. Unfortunately, the healing properties of bone broth cannot be developed with just vegetables. Although this recipe features the base ingredients for vegetable broth, I recommend adding high-quality roasted chicken or beef bones to maximize the health benefits. Allowing bones to simmer in a flavorful stock for several hours will help develop a rich, flavorful broth that contains valuable healing nutrients, minerals, and collagen. **MAKES 12 CUPS**

4 pounds roasted
   animal bones
   (optional)

3 carrots,
   roughly chopped

3 celery stalks,
   roughly chopped

1 white onion,
   roughly chopped

1 leek, white parts only,
   roughly chopped

2 garlic cloves,
   roughly chopped

½ teaspoon dried
   rosemary

1 teaspoon dried thyme

1 tablespoon dried sage

2 bay leaves

1 teaspoon salt

1 teaspoon apple
   cider vinegar

12 cups filtered water

**MAKE-AHEAD
ONE-POT**

Prep time: 15 minutes
Cook time: 6 to 20 hours

Cooking Tip: You can simmer this broth in a stockpot instead of a slow cooker if desired—just don't leave the pot unattended.

1. If using, place the roasted animal bones in the bottom of a slow cooker (see Cooking Tip).

2. Add the carrots, celery, onion, leek, garlic, rosemary, thyme, sage, bay leaves, and salt. Finally, add the apple cider vinegar and water.

3. Cook on high for 2 hours.

4. Reduce the heat to low. Allow your broth to cook anywhere from 6 to 20 hours.

5. Once it is cooked to your desired color and flavor, strain the liquid through a fine-mesh sieve into a large Mason jar or other airtight container. Discard or compost any scraps.

Recipe Tip: The longer you cook the broth, the more the flavor and color will deepen, and the more nutrients will be extracted. If you are using quality animal bones that contain a lot of collagen, your broth should gel when cooled. For the most collagen-rich options, use neck bones, shanks, and knuckles for beef or lamb; feet, wings, and neck for poultry; and neck, hock, and feet for pork. Note that the broth is still delicious and nutritious even if it doesn't gel.

Per Serving (1 cup): Calories: 20; Total Fat: 0g; Saturated Fat: 0g; Sodium: 194mg; Carbohydrates: 4g; Fiber: 1g; Protein: 1g

Bone Broth Brown Gravy

Bone broth gets its healing properties from the collagen and nutrients extracted from animal bones during the long cooking process. Collagen, the most abundant protein in the body, is said to help with many issues, from alleviating joint pain to improving skin health. **MAKES 4 SERVINGS**

3 tablespoons cassava flour

1 tablespoon extra-virgin olive oil

3 cups beef bone broth (or Homemade Vegetable Bone Broth, page 162)

5-INGREDIENT
30-MINUTE

Prep time: 5 minutes
Cook time: 20 minutes

1. In a small bowl, stir together the cassava flour and olive oil to make a roux.

2. In a small saucepan, bring the broth to a boil.

3. Once the broth is boiling, stir in the roux. Return to a boil.

4. Reduce the heat to low and simmer for 20 minutes, stirring occasionally, until the gravy thickens to your liking.

Per Serving (2 tablespoons): Calories: 79; Total Fat: 4g; Saturated Fat: 1g; Sodium: 233mg; Carbohydrates: 8g; Fiber: 1g; Protein: 5g

Ingredient Tip: You can swap out beef bone broth for chicken or turkey bone broth to make a chicken or turkey gravy.

Serving Tip: Enjoy this gravy over Baked Carrot Meatloaf (page 129) or Stuffed Cabbage Rolls (page 127).

Homemade Stir-Fry Sauce

This pantry staple adds an Asian flair to any dish. One of the most common ingredients in Asian cooking is soy sauce, which contains soy and wheat products. Thankfully, coconut liquid aminos, derived from coconut sap, is an excellent AIP-friendly substitute with a similar flavor, texture, and consistency.

MAKES 12 OUNCES

½ cup Homemade Vegetable Bone Broth (page 162) or water

½ cup coconut liquid aminos

2 tablespoons cassava flour

1 tablespoon minced garlic

1 tablespoon freshly squeezed lime juice

2 teaspoons grated peeled fresh gingerroot

1 teaspoon coconut sugar

30-MINUTE
MAKE-AHEAD
ONE-BOWL

Prep time: 5 minutes

Cooking Tip: Try this sauce with Chicken Egg Roll in a Bowl (page 105) or Bok Choy Pork Stir-Fry (page 120).

Make-Ahead Tip: You can double this recipe as needed. Store it in the refrigerator for 7 to 10 days.

1. In a Mason jar or other container with a tight-fitting lid, combine the broth, coconut aminos, flour, garlic, lime juice, ginger, and coconut sugar.

2. Seal and shake vigorously for 60 seconds, or until all ingredients are well incorporated.

Per Serving (2 ounces): Calories: 34; Total Fat: 0g; Saturated Fat: 0g; Sodium: 33mg; Carbohydrates: 7g; Fiber: 0g; Protein: 0g

Cauliflower Alfredo Sauce

Cauliflower is one of the most popular and versatile health foods out there today, and making luscious sauce out of cauliflower purée is an emerging trend within the dairy-free community. This nutrient-dense food contains almost every vita-min and mineral that the body needs. **MAKES 2 CUPS**

1 cup puréed
   cauliflower
2 tablespoons
   nutritional yeast

1 teaspoon chopped
   fresh parsley
½ teaspoon
   garlic powder
½ teaspoon salt

5-INGREDIENT
30-MINUTE
MAKE-AHEAD
ONE-POT

Prep time: 10 minutes
Cook time: 10 minutes

1. In a small saucepan over medium heat, combine the puréed cauliflower, nutritional yeast, parsley, garlic powder, and salt. Stir well.

2. Cook, stirring occasionally, until the sauce is warmed through, about 5 minutes.

Per Serving (½ cup): Calories: 35; Total Fat: 1g; Saturated Fat: 0g; Sodium: 296mg; Carbohydrates: 4g; Fiber: 2g; Protein: 4g

Cooking Tip: Add a tablespoon or two of Homemade Vegetable Bone Broth (page 162) or coconut milk to thin the sauce out if desired.

Ingredient Tip: You may be able to find puréed cauliflower in the frozen section of your local grocery store. To make your own, simply steam 3 cups of cauliflower florets and then blend or purée in a food processor until smooth.

Make-Ahead Tip: The sauce can be frozen in individual portions in ice cube trays for future use.

Chimichurri Sauce

Chimichurri is a delicious uncooked sauce that doubles as a marinade for meats, fish, and vegetables. Cilantro, one of the main ingredients, is one of the most popular herbs in the world to grow and cook with. With its powerful aroma and vibrant green color, this herb also provides many nutritional benefits. Cilantro has been used for hundreds of years, both medicinally and in culinary applications, and contains natural antioxidant and antibacterial properties.

MAKES 1½ CUPS

6 garlic cloves

¼ cup roughly chopped red onion

1½ cups fresh parsley leaves, packed

½ cup fresh cilantro leaves, packed

2 tablespoons freshly squeezed lime juice

1 tablespoon red wine vinegar

1 teaspoon salt

1 teaspoon minced peeled fresh gingerroot

30-MINUTE
MAKE-AHEAD
ONE-BOWL

Prep time: 10 minutes

1. In a food processor, pulse the garlic and red onion for 15 seconds.

2. Add the parsley, cilantro, lime juice, vinegar, salt, and ginger and process on high for 1 minute, or until smooth.

Per Serving (1 tablespoon): Calories: 4; Total Fat: 0g; Saturated Fat: 0g; Sodium: 99mg; Carbohydrates: 1g; Fiber: 0g; Protein: 0g

Make-Ahead Tip: You can make this recipe in batches, doubling it as needed. Store in the refrigerator for 7 to 10 days or freeze in ice cube trays for future use. The sauce can be frozen for up to 3 months.

Mango Agrodolce

Agrodolce is an Italian sweet-and-sour sauce. In this recipe, the sweet comes from mango and the sour comes from balsamic vinegar. Mangos contain more than 20 different vitamins and minerals, making them a delicious superfood.

MAKES 2 CUPS

1 pound ripe mangos, peeled, pitted, and diced

¾ cup white balsamic vinegar

½ cup diced yellow onion

¼ cup coconut sugar

2 teaspoons extra-virgin olive oil

2 teaspoons minced garlic

½ teaspoon salt

5-INGREDIENT
MAKE-AHEAD
ONE-POT

Prep time: 10 minutes
Cook time: 1 hour

1. In a medium saucepan, combine the mangos, vinegar, onion, sugar, oil, garlic, and salt. Place over medium-high heat and bring the mixture to a boil.

2. Allow to boil for 1 minute, stirring constantly. Reduce the heat to low and simmer for 1 hour, stirring occasionally.

3. Using an immersion blender, carefully purée until smooth. (If you don't have an immersion blender, carefully transfer the contents of the pan to a regular blender and purée until smooth, covering the top of the blender with a towel to protect yourself from hot spatters.)

4. Store the sauce in a Mason jar or other airtight container in the refrigerator.

Per Serving (½ cup): Calories: 150; Total Fat: 3g; Saturated Fat: 0g; Sodium: 295mg; Carbohydrates: 31g; Fiber: 2g; Protein: 1g

Make-Ahead Tip: Store the sauce in the refrigerator for up to 14 days or freeze in ice cube trays for individual-size portions that can be used as needed.

Ingredient Tip: Agrodolce sauce is versatile and pairs well with many cuts of meat and vegetable-based dishes. For a fresh seafood twist, try the Mahi-Mahi with Mango Agrodolce (page 78).

Sweet Beet Vinaigrette

This sweet and savory vinaigrette is perfect for topping your favorite salad or enjoying on your favorite roasted vegetables. Drawing its beautiful color from all-natural beets, this vinaigrette packs in important nutrients like fiber, folate, and naturally occurring beneficial nitrates that have been shown to help reduce blood pressure. **MAKES 12 OUNCES**

2 small cooked beets, peeled and diced

¼ cup apple cider vinegar

1 teaspoon minced garlic

1 teaspoon raw honey

½ teaspoon salt

½ teaspoon ground cinnamon

¾ cup extra-virgin olive oil

5-INGREDIENT
30-MINUTE
ONE-BOWL

Prep time: 10 minutes

1. Combine the beets, vinegar, garlic, honey, salt, and cinnamon in a tall, wide-mouth container.

2. Use an immersion blender to blend the ingredients together (see Cooking Tip).

3. With the blender running, slowly drizzle in the olive oil to emulsify.

Per Serving (2 tablespoons): Calories: 238; Total Fat: 25g; Saturated Fat: 4g; Sodium: 220mg; Carbohydrates: 5g; Fiber: 1g; Protein: 1g

Cooking Tip: Though an immersion blender is helpful here, it's okay if you don't have one. Simply combine all the ingredients in a container with a tight-fitting lid, such as a Mason jar, and shake vigorously to combine.

Substitution Tip: To make this recipe vegan-friendly, omit the honey and substitute 1 teaspoon pure maple syrup.

Apple Cider Vinaigrette

This classic pantry staple is made with simple ingredients like apple cider vinegar and olive oil. Olive oil, the natural oil extracted from the olive fruit, is predominantly composed of the monounsaturated fatty acid oleic acid, which is known for its beneficial heart health and anti-inflammatory properties.

MAKES 12 OUNCES

¼ cup apple
   cider vinegar
1 tablespoon
   minced garlic
1 tablespoon
   minced shallot

1 teaspoon raw honey
½ teaspoon salt
¾ cup extra-virgin
   olive oil

5-INGREDIENT
30-MINUTE
ONE-BOWL

Prep time: 10 minutes

1. Combine the vinegar, garlic, shallot, honey, and salt in a tall, wide-mouth container.

2. Blend the ingredients together with an immersion blender (see Cooking Tip).

3. With the blender running, slowly drizzle in the olive oil to emulsify.

Per Serving (2 tablespoons): Calories: 225; Total Fat: 25g; Saturated Fat: 4g; Sodium: 195mg; Carbohydrates: 2g; Fiber: 0g; Protein: 0g

Cooking Tip: Though an immersion blender is helpful here, it's okay if you don't have one. Simply combine all the ingredients in a container with a tight-fitting lid, such as a Mason jar, and shake vigorously to combine.

Substitution Tip: To make this recipe vegan-friendly, omit the honey and substitute 1 teaspoon pure maple syrup.

Green Goddess Dressing

This version of green goddess dressing is a bit more approachable than the original version that features mayonnaise and anchovies. Though most commonly used as a salad dressing, it can also double as a thick and creamy dip, perfect for enjoying with chopped vegetables or as a condiment for burgers and sandwiches.

MAKES ABOUT 2 CUPS

2 cups diced avocado

½ cup fresh parsley leaves, packed

½ cup light coconut milk

2 tablespoons freshly squeezed lemon juice

2 tablespoons white vinegar

1 tablespoon extra-virgin olive oil

1 tablespoon chopped fresh dill

½ teaspoon salt

30-MINUTE
MAKE-AHEAD
ONE-BOWL

Prep time: 10 minutes

Make-Ahead Tip: Store in a sealed Mason jar in the refrigerator for up to 7 days.

Ingredient Tip: You can substitute 1 teaspoon dried dill if you don't have fresh dill.

1. Add the avocado, parsley, coconut milk, lemon juice, vinegar, olive oil, dill, and salt to a food processor.

2. Blend on high for 30 to 60 seconds, or until smooth.

Per Serving (1 tablespoon): Calories: 19; Total Fat: 2g; Saturated Fat: 0g; Sodium: 25mg; Carbohydrates: 1g; Fiber: 0g; Protein: 0g

Creamy Ranch Dressing

A good dressing can make any salad or veggie taste amazing. Luckily, one of the most popular dressings today, classic ranch dressing, can be made with nutritious ingredients like fresh herbs, such as parsley, chives, and dill, which are AIP-approved. Studies have shown that parsley can aid the the body's natural detoxification pathways and may even help improve immune function.

MAKES 1 CUP

2 tablespoons chopped
    fresh chives

1 tablespoon chopped
    fresh parsley

1 tablespoon chopped
    fresh dill

1 tablespoon water

1 tablespoon
    garlic powder

1½ teaspoons
    onion powder

½ teaspoon
    white vinegar

1 cup Creamy
    Coconut Milk Yogurt
    (page 177)

30-MINUTE
MAKE-AHEAD
ONE-BOWL

Prep time: 10 minutes

Make-Ahead Tip: Refrigerate the dressing in a Mason jar or container with a tight-fitting lid for up to 7 days.

Ingredient Tip: Though you can enjoy this dressing right away, its flavors are best after being refrigerated for 6 to 12 hours.

1. Combine the chives, parsley, and dill in a food processor and pulse for 15 seconds.

2. Add the water, garlic powder, onion powder, and vinegar and pulse for 15 seconds.

3. Add the coconut milk yogurt and blend on high for 30 to 60 seconds, or until smooth.

4. Refrigerate until ready to serve (see Ingredient Tip).

Per Serving (2 tablespoons): Calories: 65; Total Fat: 6g; Saturated Fat: 11g; Sodium: 4mg; Carbohydrates: 4g; Fiber: 0g; Protein: 0g

Garlic Olive Tapenade

Tapenade is a French paste made from olives that can be enjoyed as a dip or spread, or as a stuffing for poultry or pork dishes. Olives are technically a fruit, belonging to the drupe category, similar to other stone fruits. All varieties of olives contain many health benefits, including heart-healthy fats and powerful antioxidants like the protective vitamin E. Although olives are most commonly used to make olive oil, they are very tasty on their own and offer a unique flavor profile to almost any dish. **MAKES 2½ CUPS**

4 garlic cloves

6 ounces pitted black olives

6 ounces pitted green olives

6 ounces pitted kalamata olives

3 tablespoons freshly squeezed lemon juice

2 tablespoons extra-virgin olive oil

1 tablespoon chopped fresh basil

¼ teaspoon ground oregano

30-MINUTE
MAKE-AHEAD
ONE-BOWL

Prep time: 10 minutes

1. In a food processor, pulse the garlic for 30 seconds.

2. Add the olives, lemon juice, olive oil, basil, and oregano and process until the desired consistency is achieved (see Cooking Tip).

Per Serving (2 ounces): Calories: 80; Total Fat: 8g; Saturated Fat: 1g; Sodium: 451mg; Carbohydrates: 4g; Fiber: 2g; Protein: 1g

Cooking Tip: For a chunkier tapenade, process the ingredients in step 2 for just a short time. This texture is great for salads or sandwiches. For a smoother tapenade—great for dipping veggies or spreading on AIP-Friendly Flatbread (page 176)—process the mixture for a longer time.

Make-Ahead Tip: You can make this in advance and store it in a sealed Mason jar in the refrigerator for up to 2 weeks.

Grain-Free Tortillas

Cassava flour, made from the yuca root, provides a popular staple alternative for those following a grain-free, gluten-free diet. Very mild in flavor, cassava flour is not gritty or grainy, but rather powdery like traditional flour. These grain-free tortillas may become your new favorite diet go-to. **MAKES 6 TORTILLAS**

¾ cup cassava flour,
    plus more for dusting
½ teaspoon
    garlic powder
¼ teaspoon salt

2 tablespoons
    extra-virgin olive oil
½ cup warm water
Olive oil cooking spray

5-INGREDIENT
30-MINUTE
MAKE-AHEAD

Prep time: 15 minutes
Cook time: 5 minutes.

1. In a medium bowl, whisk together the cassava flour, garlic powder, and salt.

2. Add the olive oil, followed by the water, and mix with a spatula until a dough forms. Once the mixture is thick enough, transfer the dough to a clean surface dusted with cassava flour, and knead the dough until well combined.

3. Divide the dough into 6 evenly sized portions, and roll them into balls.

4. Place each dough ball between two sheets of parchment paper and, using a rolling pin, roll it out into as thin a round as a traditional flour tortilla.

Make-Ahead Tip: Double or quadruple this recipe to make tortillas in bulk. Refrigerated tortillas will last approximately 7 days. Alternatively, layer tortillas between individual sheets of parchment paper and freeze them for up to 3 months.

5. Heat a dry nonstick skillet over medium-high heat.

6. Add 1 dough round to the dry skillet and cook for 2 to 3 minutes, or until bubbles begin to form on top and the bottom is lightly browned.

7. Flip the tortilla and cook it for an additional 2 to 3 minutes. Transfer to a plate and set aside.

8. Repeat steps 6 and 7 with the remaining dough rounds.

   Recipe Tip: To make tortilla chips, cut the tortillas into sixths and arrange the pieces on a foil-lined baking sheet. Spray with olive oil cooking spray and salt to taste and bake at 350°F for 10 minutes. Serve baked tortilla chips with Lemon Parsnip Hummus (page 49), Beet and Mango Salsa (page 50), or my personal favorite, Chimichurri Sauce (page 167).

Per Serving (1 tortilla): Calories: 60; Total Fat: 1g; Saturated Fat: 0g; Sodium: 161mg; Carbohydrates: 12g; Fiber: 2g; Protein: 0g

AIP-Friendly Flatbread

Baking while following the autoimmune protocol is very difficult because many of the traditional flours and additives like baking powder are off-limits. This AIP-friendly variation on flatbread may not be exactly the same as the traditional kind made with wheat flour, but it does a good job of providing the comforting feeling of warm bread fresh from the oven. **MAKES 4 FLATBREADS**

½ cup coconut flour
¼ cup tapioca flour
⅛ teaspoon salt
¾ cup full-fat
   coconut milk

½ teaspoon coconut oil
   or olive oil cooking
   spray, plus more
   as needed

5-INGREDIENT

30-MINUTE

Prep time: 5 minutes
Cook time: 10 minutes

1. In a large bowl, whisk together the coconut flour, tapioca flour, and salt. Pour in the coconut milk and stir until well combined.

2. Heat the coconut oil in a skillet over medium heat.

3. Add one-quarter of the batter, flattening it out to a flatbread shape and size, and cook it for 2 to 3 minutes.

4. Flip the flatbread, reduce the heat to low, and cook for another 2 to 3 minutes, or until golden brown on the outside.

5. Repeat steps 3 and 4 with the remaining dough, adding more coconut oil as necessary.

Ingredient Tip: Use this flatbread as the base for sandwiches or pizza, like Mediterranean Chicken Pizzas (page 102).

Per Serving (1 flatbread): Calories: 197; Total Fat: 13g; Saturated Fat: 11g; Sodium: 589mg; Carbohydrates: 19g; Fiber: 7g; Protein: 3g

Creamy Coconut Milk Yogurt

The absence of dairy in the AIP may leave some feeling like they are missing key components of cooking, including items like yogurt and cream for sauces and other dishes. Thankfully, yogurt can be made at home using the same traditional method of combining liquid with cultures, or bacteria. This leads to fermentation, in which the bacteria converts the sugar into lactic acid, giving the yogurt its trademark thickness and tang. **MAKES 4 SERVINGS**

1 (14-ounce) can full-fat coconut milk

2 high-quality probiotic capsules (see Ingredient Tip)

5-INGREDIENT ONE-BOWL

Prep time: 10 minutes
Cook time: 48 hours

1. Sterilize a Mason jar or other glass container with a tight-fitting lid by submerging it in boiling water (see Cooking Tip).

2. Add the coconut milk to the sterilized jar, seal the jar, and shake until well combined and smooth.

3. Carefully twist the probiotic capsules until the end caps come apart, and sprinkle the contents into the jar.

4. Seal the jar, then shake vigorously until well combined.

5. Allow the closed jar to sit on the counter for 24 to 48 hours to allow fermentation to begin. Shake occasionally.

6. After 24 to 48 hours, put the jar in the refrigerator. This will allow the mixture to thicken to your desired consistency.

7. Refrigerate for up to 7 days.

Ingredient Tip: The probiotic capsule will make or break this recipe. You want a high-quality capsule that contains probiotics in the billions, ranging from 10 to 50 billion. Double-check that your capsule does not have any other added ingredients or prebiotics.

Cooking Tip: Sterilizing your container will kill any bacteria that may potentially infiltrate your yogurt.

Per Serving (½ cup): Calories: 230; Total Fat: 24g; Saturated Fat: 21g; Sodium: 15mg; Carbohydrates: 6g; Fiber: 2g; Protein: 2g

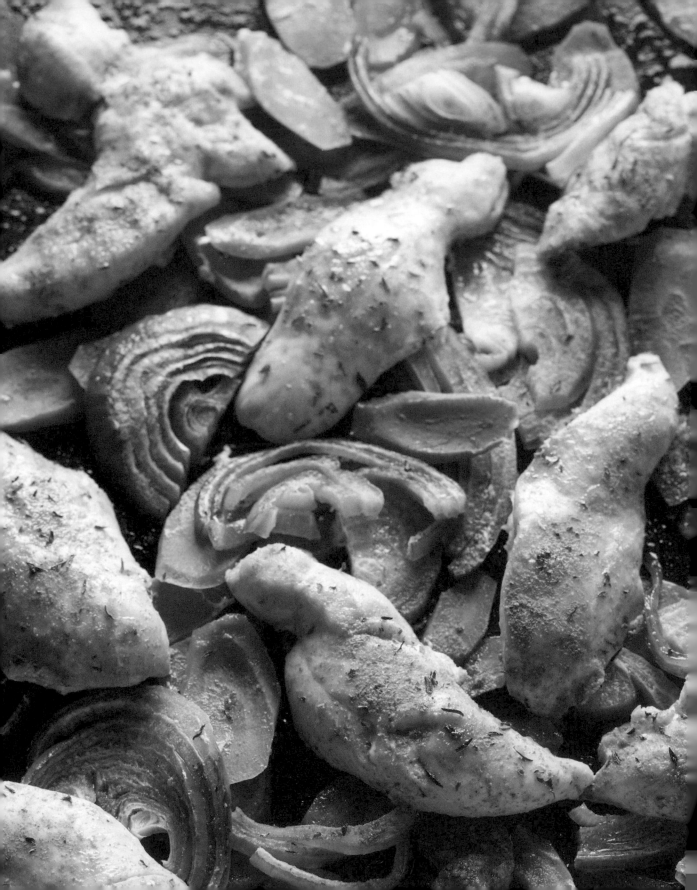

How to Reintroduce Foods

After you complete the elimination phase of the paleo autoimmune protocol, it can be both exciting and nerve-wracking to start the reintroduction phase. One of the most common questions I get from my clients is, "How do I know when I can start reintroducing foods?" I recommend that my clients follow the elimination phase of the protocol for a minimum of 30 days before attempting any reintroductions. On top of that, I want to see that there has been a positive improvement in the management of unwanted symptoms *before* any eliminated foods are added back to the diet. If you have been following the elimination phase for 30 days and have still not seen the improvements you were hoping for, I recommend following the protocol for another two weeks while also working closely with your health care practitioner to ensure that any potential underlying problems are addressed.

If, after 30 days, you feel that you have seen a positive and dramatic reduction in your most unwanted symptoms, you are likely ready to start the reintroduction phase of the protocol. During the reintroduction phase, it is critical that you proceed with caution—this is not a time to start eating anything and everything. The reintroduction phase is just as strict as the elimination phase and requires just as much planning and dedication, if not more, to execute effectively. This is a time of learning and exploring, when you will discover which foods are your biggest triggers so you can begin to create the most liberal, personalized, anti-inflammatory protocol customized to your own unique needs. During this phase I recommend using a symptom tracker (page 182) to track the foods you have consumed and any associated symptoms. This will allow you to monitor your progress and collect valuable data for your continuing treatment plan.

There are many different ways to approach food reintroduction. The most effective and impactful reintroduction schedule is the longest and most time consuming, but it is also most likely to yield the greatest results. This method involves testing a small amount of each new food for three days, and then, if there are no negative reactions, testing a large amount of the new food for three more days. This process is designed to detect both immediate and delayed hypersensitivity reactions, since some foods can cause negative reactions up to 72 hours after consumption. Additionally, many hypersensitivity reactions are dose-related, meaning that a small amount may not produce unwanted symptoms, but a large amount will. In a perfect world, foods should be reintroduced following a schedule like this one (using egg yolk as the example food), which accounts for both delayed reactions and dose-related reactions:

Day 1: Eat a small amount of the untested food—for this example, half of a cooked egg yolk.

Days 1 to 3: Monitor your body for two or three days for any unwanted signs and symptoms. If you do not experience any negative reactions, move on to day 4. If you do experience any negative reactions, record them appropriately in your symptom tracker (page 182) and make a note that egg yolks will remain on your eliminated foods list.

Day 4: If you have not experienced a negative reaction since eating the half egg yolk on day 1, now it's time to try a larger test dose—for this example, three cooked egg yolks.

Days 4 to 6: Monitor your body for two or three days for any unwanted signs and symptoms. If you do not experience any negative reactions, continue to enjoy this food in your diet. If you do experience any negative reactions, record them appropriately in your symptom tracker and remove the food completely from your diet.

Following this reintroduction method means that a new food will be tested every six days, and I recommend that my clients only attempt one new food per week. Of course, this is not always feasible. Many of my clients resort to shorter food reintroduction schedules, waiting just one or two days between trials. However, this accelerated method is not ideal because it may make it harder to pinpoint associated symptoms down the road. Ultimately, the best process for you will take into account physical, mental, emotional, and social aspects of real, everyday life. You may even consider working one-on-one with a trained health care professional during this stage of the protocol, as they can offer guidance and draw on their experience to create a unique plan tailored to your lifestyle and symptoms.

Now that we've covered the framework of a food reintroduction schedule, the next step is to determine which foods should be reintroduced first. The following suggested order of food reintroductions was created by the Paleo Mom, Dr. Sarah Ballantyne, based on the likelihood that each food will cause a reaction (in order from least likely to most likely):

1. Egg yolks
2. Grass-fed ghee
3. Seed-derived spices
4. Legumes (except soy)
5. Nuts
6. Seeds
7. Nightshades (except tomatoes)
8. Coffee
9. Chocolate

Of course, this list is not all encompassing and will look different for each individual. Work with your health care provider to create a customized reintroduction schedule that works best for you and your current situation. At this point you should continue to avoid gluten, dairy, and soy, as well as any foods you already suspect or know cause sensitivity or allergic reactions. Over time, this process should allow you to create a highly customized anti-inflammatory protocol that is unique to you and your own dietary triggers.

Completing the reintroduction phase as methodically and patiently as possible is the key to ensuring you are getting the most out of the hard work that you put in during the elimination phase of the AIP. The goal is to be able to identify which foods trigger your reactions, eliminate them, and enjoy the other foods you know to be "safe" and healthy for your body. Again, the point is not to live on a severely restricted diet forever, but rather to be free from perceived restrictions and enjoy a variety of foods as safely as possible. Having a well thought-out plan ahead of time is important, and using a symptom tracker is critical for gathering data that will help you create your own customized plan.

Symptom Tracker

Use this page to track symptoms. Make as many copies as you need so you can continue to track symptoms as you reintroduce foods.

DATE	FOOD REINTRODUCED	AMOUNT	SYMPTOMS	DESIGNATION (Okay, Limit, Avoid)

Measurement Conversions

	US STANDARD	US STANDARD (OUNCES)	METRIC (APPROXIMATE)
VOLUME EQUIVALENTS (LIQUID)	2 tablespoons	1 fl. oz.	30 mL
	¼ cup	2 fl. oz.	60 mL
	½ cup	4 fl. oz.	120 mL
	1 cup	8 fl. oz.	240 mL
	1 ½ cups	12 fl. oz.	355 mL
	2 cups or 1 pint	16 fl. oz.	475 mL
	4 cups or 1 quart	32 fl. oz.	1 L
	1 gallon	128 fl. oz.	4 L
VOLUME EQUIVALENTS (DRY)	⅛ teaspoon		0.5 mL
	¼ teaspoon		1 mL
	½ teaspoon		2 mL
	¾ teaspoon		4 mL
	1 teaspoon		5 mL
	1 tablespoon		15 mL
	¼ cup		59 mL
	⅓ cup		79 mL
	½ cup		118 mL
	⅔ cup		156 mL
	¾ cup		177 mL
	1 cup		235 mL
	2 cups or 1 pint		475 mL
	3 cups		700 mL
	4 cups or 1 quart		1 L
	½ gallon		2 L
	1 gallon		4 L
WEIGHT EQUIVALENTS	½ ounce		15 g
	1 ounce		30 g
	2 ounces		60 g
	4 ounces		115 g
	8 ounces		225 g
	12 ounces		340 g
	16 ounces or 1 pound		455 g

Resources

WEBSITES

Emily Kyle Nutrition (emilykylenutrition.com): Blog and website from author Emily Kyle, focusing on holistic health care for autoimmune and inflammatory conditions. Here you'll find many free resources, evidence-based nutrition-related articles, and Hashimoto's- and AIP-friendly recipes.

Thyroid Awareness (thyroidawareness.com): Website from The American Association of Clinical Endocrinologists. Contains updated information regarding thyroid conditions and the types of treatments available, plus downloadable/printable resources.

The American Thyroid Association (thyroid.org): Resources from the leading organization devoted to thyroid biology and the prevention and treatment of thyroid disease.

The Invisible Hypothyroidism (theinvisiblehypothyroidism.com): Website created by thyroid patient expert and advocate Rachel Hill. Provides a realistic, compassionate, and knowledgeable perspective on living and thriving with thyroid conditions.

The Paleo Mom (thepaleomom.com): Website created by medical biophysicist and mom Sarah Ballantyne, PhD. Includes family-friendly recipes, practical tips, and detailed articles about how diet and lifestyle impact health.

Autoimmune Wellness (autoimmunewellness.com): Resources specific to the healing journey of autoimmune sufferers.

Simply AIP (simplyaip.com): Website for monthly delivery subscription service that includes grab-and-go snacks, sweet treats, AIP pantry staples, recipes, self-care tips, and online community support.

BOOKS

The 30-Minute Thyroid Cookbook: 125 Healing Recipes for Hypothyroidism & Hashimoto's, by Emily Kyle, MS, RDN, CDN, CLT (Rockridge Press, 2018)

The Autoimmune Solution: Prevent and Reverse the Full Spectrum of Inflammatory Symptoms and Diseases, by Amy Myers, MD (HarperOne, 2017)

Hashimoto's Protocol: A 90-Day Plan for Reversing Thyroid Symptoms and Getting Your Life Back, by Izabella Wentz, PhD (HarperOne, 2017)

Why Do I Still Have Thyroid Symptoms? When My Lab Tests Are Normal: A Revolutionary Breakthrough in Understanding Hashimoto's Disease and Hypothyroidism, by Dr. Datis Kharrazian (Elephant Press, 2010)

Be Your Own Thyroid Advocate: When You're Sick and Tired of Being Sick and Tired, by Rachel Hill (independently published, 2018)

The Medical Medium, Thyroid Healing, by Anthony William (Hay House Inc., 2017)

References

"Autoimmune Diseases." National Institute of Arthritis and Musculoskeletal and Skin Diseases, U.S. Department of Health and Human Services. Accessed March 1, 2019. www.niams.nih.gov/health-topics/autoimmune-diseases.

"Autoimmune Diseases." U.S. Department of Health & Human Services Office on Women's Health, October 2018. www.womenshealth.gov/a-z-topics /autoimmune-diseases.

Begic-Karup, S., et al. 2001. "Serum Calcium in Thyroid Disease." *The Central European Journal of Medicine* 113(1–2):65–68. https://www.ncbi.nlm.nih.gov /pubmed/11233472.

"Hashimoto's Disease." Mayo Clinic. Accessed May 13, 2019. https://www .mayoclinic.org/diseases-conditions/hashimotos-disease/symptoms-causes /syc-20351855.

"Hashimoto's Disease." U.S. Department of Health & Human Services Office on Women's Health, October 2018. www.womenshealth.gov/a-z-topics /hashimotos-disease.

"Hypothyroidism." American Thyroid Association. Accessed May 13, 2019. www .thyroid.org/hypothyroidism/.

"Iodine Deficiency." American Thyroid Association. Accessed March 9, 2019. https:// www.thyroid.org/iodine-deficiency/.

Kharrazian, Datis. "Goiter, Goitrogens, and Thyroid Enlargement." Accessed March 9, 2019. https://drknews.com/goiter-goitrogens-and-thyroid-enlargement/.

Mackawy, A.M., B.M. Al-Ayed, and B.M. Al-Rashidi. 2013. "Vitamin D Deficiency and Its Association with Thyroid Disease." *International Journal of Health Sciences* 7(3):267–275. https://www.ncbi.nlm.nih.gov/pmc/articles/PMC3921055/.

Mu, Qinghui, et al. 2017. "Leaky Gut as a Danger Signal for Autoimmune Diseases." *Frontiers in Immunology* 8 (May 27). https://doi.org/10.3389 /fimmu.2017.00598.

"Reintroductions on the Paleo AIP: The Definitive Guide." Autoimmune Wellness, July 16, 2018. autoimmunewellness.com/how-to-reintroduce-food -on-aip-the-definitive-guide/.

Somers, Emily, et al. 2009. "Are Individuals with an Autoimmune Disease at Higher Risk of a Second Autoimmune Disorder?" *American Journal of Epidemiology* 169(6):749–755. https://doi.org/10.1093/aje/kwn408.

"Symptoms of Hashimoto's Thyroiditis." EndocrineWeb. Accessed May 13, 2019. www.endocrineweb.com/conditions/hashimotos-thyroiditis/symptoms -hashimotos-thyroiditis.

Index

Acknowledgments

If you're wondering why all of the recipes in this book taste so good, it is
100 percent because of the true talent of my husband, Chef Phil. He put a tremendous amount of time, energy, and dedication into the creation of this cookbook.
Although the autoimmune protocol was completely new to him, he took on the
challenge of creating delicious, chef-quality recipes with limited ingredients. We
both learned a lot together, and we even surprised ourselves with how good some
of our own creations turned out.

Chef Phil, you have been my greatest fan these past nine years. You have encouraged
me to follow my dreams time and time again, and together we make the perfect team.
I love you. Thank you for all that you do for me, and thank you for the magic you have
brought to this cookbook.

And to my four-year old son, Ransom, the one who spends long days in the
kitchen with me, you truly are my best friend. Thank you for your patience as
Mommy finishes another book—soon we will celebrate at Disney World.

About the Authors

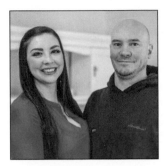

Emily Kyle is an award-winning, nationally recognized media dietitian, nutrition spokesperson, and published author. She is the owner of Emily Kyle Nutrition (EKN), a nutrition communications and consulting company located in Rochester, NY. Through EKN, Emily offers in-person and virtual consultations and nutritional guidance with a specialty in LEAP/MRT Food Sensitivity Testing and Medical Nutrition Therapy for autoimmune and inflammatory conditions. She also practices as a Certified Holistic Cannabis Practitioner, providing evidence-based cannabis counseling and educational resources.

On her blog (*The Millennial Garden*) and social media channels, Emily shares useful resources, nutrition articles, delicious and nutritious anti-inflammatory recipes, and her passion for backyard gardening and modern homesteading. You can also catch her live every Monday on the *Good Day Rochester* morning TV show, where she demos and chats about delicious, healthy food.

Phil Kyle is a chef, successful culinary entrepreneur, and restaurant owner with more than two decades of restaurant experience. He joined the EKN team in 2019 as the executive chef and culinary director. By combining both Emily and Phil's expertise, EKN is able to deliver incredible chef-developed and -tested recipes and stunning food and lifestyle photography that both consumers and brands love, along with the clinical and nutritional knowledge of a registered dietitian.

Emily and Kyle's first book, *The 30-Minute Thyroid Cookbook: 125 Healing Recipes for Hypothyroidism & Hashimoto's*, was released in December 2018. Outside of work, you can find Emily and Phil caring for their garden, flock of chickens, and young son, Ransom.